SECRETS TO A HEALTHY KIDNEY

A Common Man's Guide

DR MURUGANANTH SUBRAMANIAM

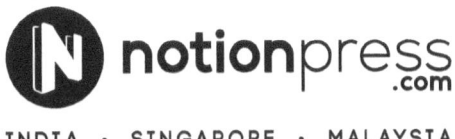

INDIA • SINGAPORE • MALAYSIA

Notion Press Media Pvt Ltd

No. 50, Chettiyar Agaram Main Road,
Vanagaram, Chennai, Tamil Nadu – 600 095

First Published by Notion Press 2021
Copyright © Dr Murugananth Subramaniam 2021
All Rights Reserved.

ISBN 978-1-63745-375-9

This book has been published with all efforts taken to make the material error-free after the consent of the author. However, the author and the publisher do not assume and hereby disclaim any liability to any party for any loss, damage, or disruption caused by errors or omissions, whether such errors or omissions result from negligence, accident, or any other cause.

While every effort has been made to avoid any mistake or omission, this publication is being sold on the condition and understanding that neither the author nor the publishers or printers would be liable in any manner to any person by reason of any mistake or omission in this publication or for any action taken or omitted to be taken or advice rendered or accepted on the basis of this work. For any defect in printing or binding the publishers will be liable only to replace the defective copy by another copy of this work then available.

Contents

Foreword 5
Preface 13
Acknowledgements 15

Part 1. Basic Facts and Diseases Affecting the Kidneys 17

    Autobiography of the Kidney 18
    Kidney Disease – Symptoms and Tests 24
    Kidney Disease – The Real Problem 31
    Sugar Bites – Kidney Disease in Diabetes 35
    Blood Pressure and the Kidneys 41
    Kidney Stones 47
    How Germs Attack the Kidneys? 55
    Protein Loss in Urine and Remedies 59
    Kidney Cysts 63
    Kidney Cancer 67
    Kidney Diseases in Children.. 70
    Kidney Diseases in Women 76
    As the Age Advances – Kidney Ailment in Elderly 80
    Remember, Drugs Can Do Harm to the Kidneys 84

Part 2. Kidney Failure and Treatment 89

    Kidney Attack – Acute Kidney Failure 90
    Chronic Kidney Failure 94
    When End-Stage Kidney Disease Strikes 98
    How to Postpone Dialysis? 104
    Cleansing the Blood – Dialysis 109
    Getting a New Kidney – Kidney Transplantation 119
    Kidney Beats – Getting Organ from a Brain Dead Donor 125

Part 3. What You Eat Matters! 129

    The Story of Salt 130
    Water – The Indispensable Medicine 134
    Diet You Need to Know 138
    Diet in Diabetes and Hypertension Patients 152
    Diet in Dialysis Patients 155
    Diet in Kidney Stone Disease 158
    Top 10 Super Foods 163

Part 4. Kidney Disease Prevention 171

    Exercise as Therapy 172
    Yoga, Pranayama and Meditation 176
    Heart and Kidneys 179
    Prevention is Better than Cure 181
    Protect Your Kidney from Environmental Hazards 184
    Kidney Health in Your Hands 187

Part 5. Others 191

    Kidney Warriors – 1 192
    Kidney Warriors – 2 197
    Engaging Kidney Patients and Social Responsibilities 203
    Frequently Asked Questions 205
    Common Drugs in Kidney Diseases 208
    Become an Organ Donor 211

Foreword

Chennai, India

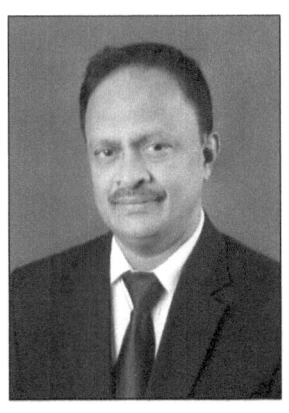

It is my great pleasure to write 'foreword' to this wonderful book on kidney and kidney diseases.

We are in an unenviable situation, with the threat of 'chronic kidney disease' looming large at an epidemic proportion and with an appalling insensitivity of the people and society about the besieging threat!

Prevailing knowledge on kidney disease among the public, is meagre, incomplete and often fraught with misconceptions. Hence, such a venture is in great need.

The book has been carefully and intelligently conceptualised to furnish a concise overview on almost all the common problems pertaining to kidney.

Though the book has been titled 'Secrets to a Healthy Kidney', it has covered the entire gamut of common kidney ailments and the treatment options.

The design of first chapter as 'monologue' by kidney itself is something innovative and sets the pace for going through the process of learning about kidney.

It is appreciable that due emphasis has been given for the two most common diseases inflicting injury on the kidney, viz. Diabetes and Hypertension.

The flow of the successive chapters is smooth and there is a fine thread of continuity. Elaboration of dialysis modalities has been done in a simple and easily understandable way without compromising on the scientific overtone. Inclusion of a chapter on measures to postpone dialysis initiation is commendable!

Information provided on diet with 'sample diet plan' for kidney failure patients will certainly serve as a ready reference for patients and treating physicians.

Inclusion of personal anecdote makes the discussion on kidney transplantation more exciting.

There are two great strengths of this book which have made it unique are emphasis on kidney health promotion and kidney disease prevention. Even the recent contentious issues like role of environmental pollution and chemicals on the causation of kidney failure have been included. The adverse effect of 'heat stress' could have been added.

And, the highlight is the sincere effort of the author to infuse confidence into the minds of the unfortunate patients upon whom the diagnosis of kidney failure has befallen as an unexpected bolt from the sky. Quite often, the much needed psychological counselling is simply not done. The author has done this with an uncanny sensitivity, quoting celebrities and achievers as examples!

Overall, this book has all the requisites to get classified as a 'Kidney Health Education' tool for public.

The simple language, reader-friendly style, comprehensiveness of information, appropriate illustrations and elegant quotes have contributed to the 'high quality' of the book.

I congratulate Dr. Murugananth for venturing and successfully accomplishing the task of authoring such a wonderful manual of kidney diseases for the public. Dr. Murugananth is well known for his academic excellence and scientific pursuits; this book has brought to surface his yet another virtue, 'social responsibility'!

My best wishes to Dr. Murugananth.

– Dr. N. Gopalakrishnan
MD DM FRCP
Director, Institute of Nephrology
Madras Medical College

Coimbatore, India

Greetings.

In today's fast paced world, we all know that there has been a significant compromise in the attention given to well-being and good health. This is compounded by the sustained increase in the adverse impacts on our body systems due to lifestyle change, pollution, diet practices, etc.

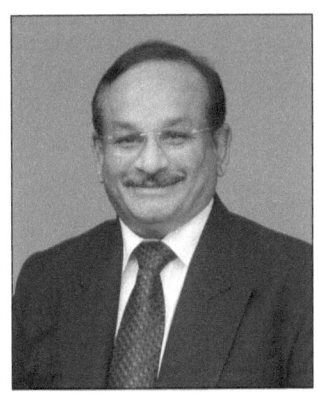

Kidney, as we all know, is an important organ in the body which helps balance the internal chemical and biochemical systems and helps excrete a significant portion of the waste generated by the routine body functions. Any disturbance in this system will lead to accumulation of the waste generated in our body which will have profound detrimental effect on the health to the extent of severe compromise of daily activity.

The most important and the first step forward to avoid and deal with health-related problems is Awareness. I find this book very simple to understand with informative content which educates about the importance of kidney function and the necessity to preserve it. Dr. S. Murugananth has made a sincere effort to ensures that sufficient knowledge is gained about common kidney problems, when to seek medical help early and measures which will preserve the kidney function.

"Secrets to a Healthy Kidney" is a comprehensive guide to Kidney awareness and is a good book to read and stay healthy.

Wishing all Good Health and Happiness...

– Dr. K. Madeswaran
Chairman & Managing Director
Consultant Neuro and Spine Surgeon
Royal Care Super Speciality Hospitals, Coimbatore

Coimbatore, India

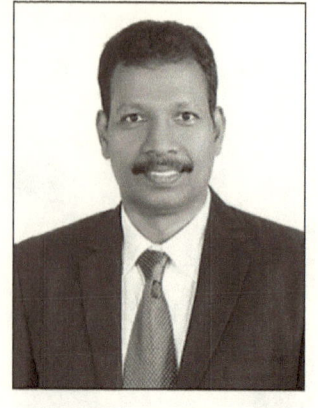

Medical health related books are intended to convey certain information to a selected audience.

"Secrets to a Healthy kidney" by Dr. S. Murugananth addresses the basic facts about kidney health and disease to the needy population, prior to a Nephrologist consultation, as a motivating book after being identified as a patient with kidney illness. The script is more of a novel and takes the audience through a model of a patient's life example the author went through in his career, then about the illness and followed by a message. Facts about diet, exercise, meditation, yoga is well highlighted. Preventive methods and the need to preserve the renal function is well described. Frequently asked questions regarding kidney illness are explained well. Real life stories of few people are a motivational experience. Quotes by leaders aptly suits the description and are remembered to the script. Its worth a read and possession.

– Dr. K. Chockalingam
Consultant Interventional Cardiologist
Royal Care Super Speciality Hospitals
Coimbatore

Attapadi, Kerala, India.

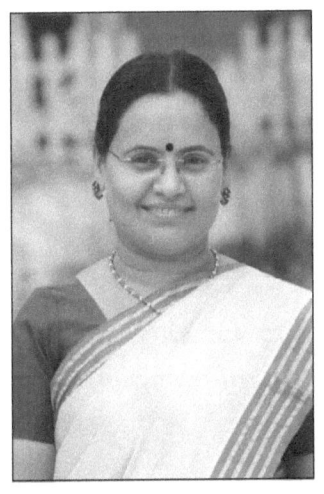

It is my privilege to introduce this book **"Secrets to a Healthy Kidney"** to every person who wants to be fit and fine. If one reads this book before interacting with the Doctor, it would be beneficial to avoid miscommunication about the diseases and will have a better understanding about the treatment. So I can confidently say this book, "SECRETS TO A HEALTHY KIDNEY" is perfectly a KNOWLEDGE BANK.

This book is to be kept in every house and every library. We have to read this kind of book along with our education and as first book when we grew up our reading habits. Through this book we can understand about consequences of the kidney diseases. If we make reading handbooks as a part of our lifestyle, we can be free from the cluster of diseases and can lead a healthy life.

My favourite part of this book is the chapter on **"Become an Organ Donor"** including the quotes of **Khalil Gibran** – *"You give but little when you give of your possessions. It is when you give of yourself that you truly give."* One can preach many things, but to make it happen is very difficult. I believe good health and good sense are two of life's greatest blessings in one's life. I donated my Kidney in the year of 1999. At that time there was no awareness about Kidney diseases, Kidney transplantation, kidney donation, etc. If a book like this was available at that time, it would have helped me much more those days.

I recommend this book to anyone who wish to be healthy, especially to Diabetic and Hypertension patients who must read and keep a copy of this book with you. When common man has more awareness they can abstain from kidney diseases or can postpone the possibility of afflicted with Kidney related issues in their life span.

Congratulations to the author of this book, my friend, Dr. Murugananth

BEST WISHES TO EVERYONE TO BE HEALTHY AND FINE.

– Uma Preman
Social Activist
Donated her kidney to a stranger in 1999
Founder – Santhi medical information centre

Hyderabad, India

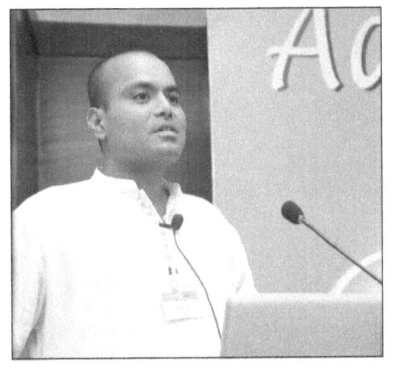

"Secrets to a Healthy Kidney" by Dr. Murugananth Subramaniam is a book that explains in simple language the functions of a kidney, the various types of kidney diseases, how to prevent them, what to do if you get them, diet to follow for various stages and types of kidney disease and most importantly, how to live well despite having kidney disease.

This book is devoid of any complex medical jargon and explains these complicated topics in a very simple, easy-to-understand manner with diagrams and quotes that add a delightful flavour to the narrative. It will be easily understood by lay people.

The book has some very useful and practical tips to prevent kidney disease and the importance of knowledge, exercise and diet in this journey.

I really liked the way many chapters began with a real life story in brief from Dr. Murugananth Subramaniam's practice which gives a nice background to the topic being discussed and brings life to each chapter.

I would recommend this book to anyone looking for more information about how to keep kidneys healthy in an easy-to-understand manner. This book is for those who would like a broad conceptual understanding of the landscape of kidney disease without being bogged down by too much detail and medical terms.

– Kamal D Shah
On dialysis since 1997
Co-founder of NephroPlus – India's largest
network of dialysis centres

Preface

"The superior doctor prevents sickness;
The mediocre doctor attends to impending sickness;
The inferior doctor treats actual sickness."

— **Proverb**

Medicine has evolved to great heaps over the last 100 years. The average life span of human being has increased by virtue of improvement in early childhood mortality. But the sick life span has increased owing to the daunting increase in many chronic diseases and kidney disease is one of them.

The global burden of kidney disease is increasing due to food and lifestyle changes. Kidney disease can strike anyone. It is important to have good knowledge of kidney diseases.

The idea of writing this book struck me on seeing many of the patients having insufficient knowledge about kidney diseases. Even those well educated have very little knowledge, which hampers them from instituting the right preventive and therapeutic measures.

I have encountered diverse patients during my period of learning and practice of nephrology. I have penned what I have conversed with them about the disease and its prevention and how they tackled the disease. This would make the readers understand better.

Knowing about kidney failure alone may not be valuable if one doesn't know about the root cause and various afflictions that would finally culminate in kidney failure. This would give a broad sense of how to go about the disease and know how not to land up in an inevitable stage. This book explains in detail on how kidneys are affected by various diseases. This would help and motivate you in the efforts of prevention from a very early stage.

The progression of kidney failure can be largely prevented, but it needs a comprehensive understanding which is most often difficult during a physician consult. This book will aid in this knowledge to a great extent.

Living a healthy and normal life after the diagnosis of end-stage kidney failure is easier than ever before. There are various options of renal replacement therapy and I have explained how to choose one. I have also given a vivid picture of its advantages and disadvantages.

Diet and lifestyle information is widely available everywhere. Here, I have given what to eat and what not, pertaining to the stage of kidney dysfunction. The information is also useful for diabetes and hypertension patients and is a must read to maintain good health. The importance of salt and water is picturised in separate chapters.

Preventive measures for kidney diseases are shockingly deficient even in developed countries. The modes of prevention and the interplay of various organs are well explained in this book and would give the readers a good road map for the same.

Many people have fought against the odds and bravely conquered kidney disease with extreme courage and perseverance. I have narrated the story of a few of them in the final chapters. This will give a clear sense of hope to the patients and the caregivers.

Not only kidney disease patients and caregivers but the general public who want to have a broad view of kidney diseases will find this book to be of great interest.

Research has shown that knowledge of the disease improves the quality of life for patients with kidney ailments and empowers one to make smart choices and take steps to achieve better health.

– Dr. Murugananth
Coimbatore
India

Acknowledgements

I pray and thank almighty God for making me what I am today.

I thank my parents, my wife, children, friends, colleagues and relatives who have guided me so far and in the course of this book.

I am indebted to my professors who taught me the Art of Medicine; Dr. V. Venugopal, Dr. S. Shivakumar, Dr. N. Gopalakrishnan and Dr. T. Balasubramaniyan without whom this book would not have been possible.

I express my gratitude to Dr. K. Madeswaran, Chairman of Royal Care Super Speciality Hospital, Coimbatore for his constant motivation and guidance.

I thank Dr. N. Gopalakrishnan, Director, Institute of Nephrology, Madras Medical College, Chennai for his valuable foreword. I pay my thanks to Dr. Madeswaran, Dr. Chockalingam, Shri. Kamal Shah and Srimathi. Uma Preman for their valuable comments for the book.

I thank Dr. Jayaprakash, Associate Professor of Nephrology, SRM Medical College, Chennai for his inputs for the book.

I thank the Notion press publishers who have accepted to publish this book.

I thank Mr. Dinesh Rajendran, Mr. Dinesh Babu and Mr. Vijay for their valuable assistance.

Last but not the least I thank all my patients who are the base of my knowledge.

PART 1

Basic Facts and Diseases Affecting the Kidneys

Autobiography of the Kidney

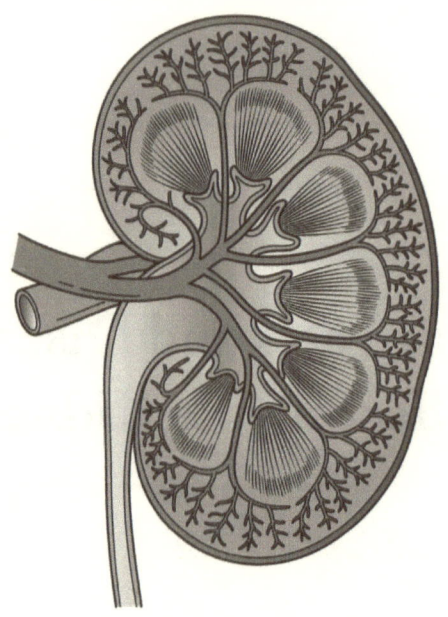

"We must acknowledge that our kidneys constitute the major foundation of our physiological freedom."

– HW Smith (Renal Physiologist)

The kidneys are extraordinary organs, It does not allow your system to poison you.

Let me speak–
I am a part of your body. I start my function even before you are born. We are twins placed on your lower back. I am very small about the size of your fist (about 10 cm long, 6 cm wide, 150-200 grams in weight.)

But please don't judge us by our size. We are capable of many more things than you would imagine.

We make up about only 150 grams each but we receive about 20% of your body's blood pumped from the heart.

Do you know how I evolved?
My growth begins at 8 weeks after the embryo develops in the mother's womb. I start producing urine in the 10th week of pregnancy. From then until death, I do my work relentlessly without expecting anything in return.

The Size of the Kidney

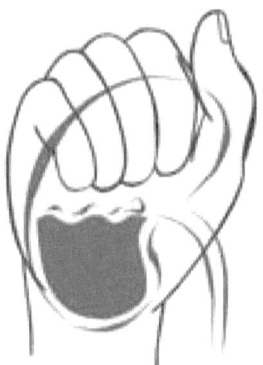

Where is the kidney?

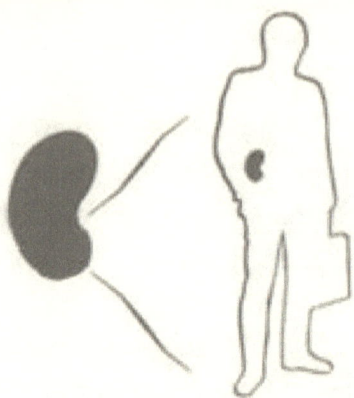

What Do We Do? (Our Functions)
Excretion of toxins

You take up food and various chemicals contained in it on a daily basis. Subsequently, chemical reactions take place in trillions of cells in the body and thousands of waste products enter into the bloodstream.

My main task is to eliminate the substances and toxins released by these events. Of these, easily quantifiable in the blood are urea and creatinine. If I don't function effectively thousands of chemicals (uremic toxins) start to accumulate in the blood.

Too much water in your body is also a toxin. Only if the water content in your body is in a balanced state, the functioning of the organs will be in order. My job is also to push out excess water out from your body.

Keeping mineral levels in a balanced state

Mineral salts such as sodium, potassium and phosphorus are present inside the cells and in the bloodstream. If the amount of such minerals in the body is too high or too low, I will expel it. I will regulate them in blood by altering their quantity in urine and thereby keeping them in a balanced state.

Blood pressure

If you add more salt to your diet, you may have high blood pressure. When I am doing well and you take a moderate amount of salt, I will keep the blood pressure in a normal range. But if you continue to consume excess salt, I have no choice but to raise the blood pressure (Hypertension) and disturb you. Only by raising the blood pressure, I can push out excess salt.

Red blood cells (Hemoglobin)

To keep the level of red blood cells adequate, I secrete a chemical substance called erythropoetin which keeps the hemoglobin at a steady level. That's why you get anemia when I don't function well.

Vitamin D

Vitamin D is produced by your body through sunlight. This vitamin is essential for functioning of all the cells of the body. I catalyse to enhance this vitamin and bring it to its full functioning capacity. When we are affected in the long term, bone pain develops due to its deficiency.

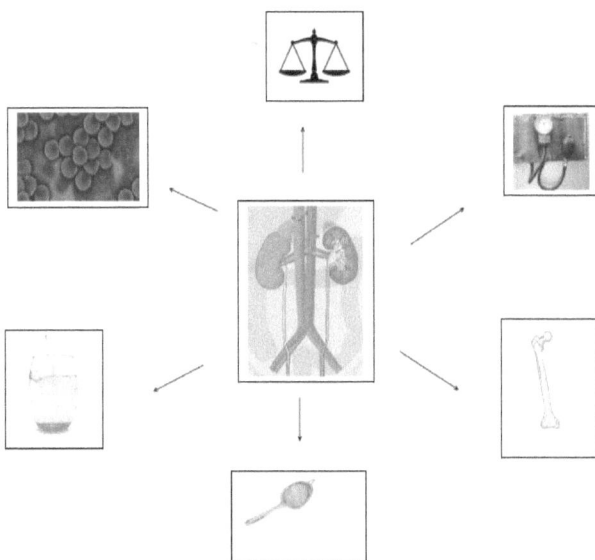

How I do these things?

The cleansing station of the body

There are about 10 lakh nephrons in each of us and all of them act as natural filters. The length of a nephron is three to five mm in size. If all the nephrons were lined up, it would be over a hundred miles.

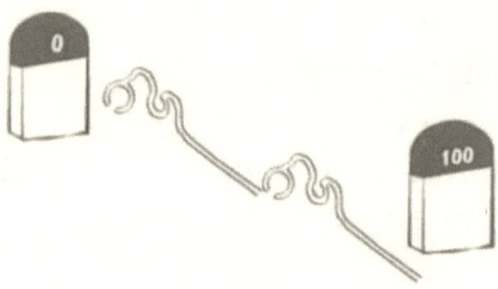

Each nephron receives blood through small blood vessels. About 125 ml of filtrate per minute is formed by us from the received blood. The mineral salts and water passes through the nephron. About 99% of the filtrate is returned to your body.

As a purification station in your body, whole blood passes through both of us about **300 times each day** to cleanse the blood repeatedly. By this, we receive about 1500 litres of blood each day, make 180 litres of filtrate, send back 99% of it and excrete the remaining 1-2 litres as urine.

Urinary Tract Structure

The resulting urine reaches the urinary bladder through the ureter. The urine is then excreted.

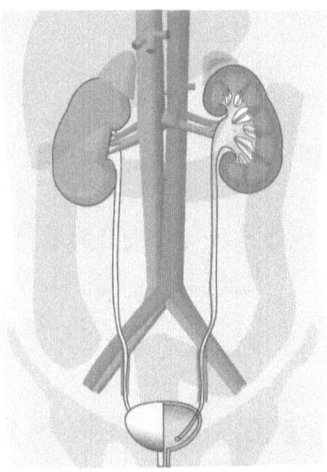

Gift of nature

Nature has given a gift to you by giving two of us. If one of us gets affected or injured, the other one takes full charge. A normal kidney can adapt and can greatly tolerate this increase in workload.

Me and pregnant mothers

Few things do harm to me in the mother's womb. Some of the pills that the mother consumes do damage to me. So, during pregnancy, have the right food and medications. If the nutrition of the fetus is affected, it may eventually affect our functioning.

*"Even with 10% of kidney function,
patients can live a normal life which is not true
with other organs, but one needs to be aware and preserve it."*

Kidney Disease – Symptoms and Tests

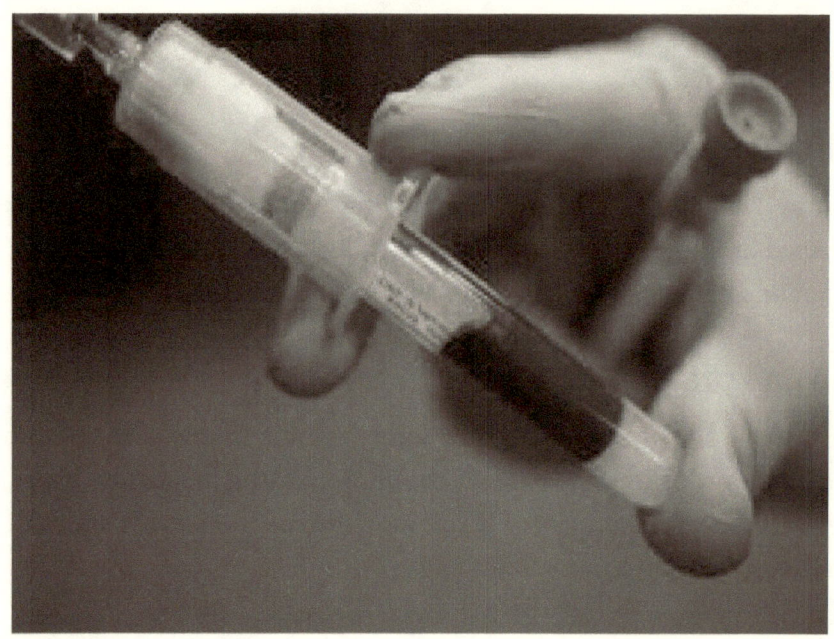

"If we make the correct diagnosis then healing can begin."

– Andrew Wolf (Physician)

We will discuss some of the symptoms and tests of kidney diseases

Swelling of Feet and Face

When fluid increases it accumulates in the loose and dependent tissues of the body. It is usually around the eyes and feet. It commonly indicates heart, kidney or liver dysfunction. It can happen also in anaemia, thyroid dysfunction or due to some pills. If the cause is not obvious your doctor may evaluate for these illnesses.

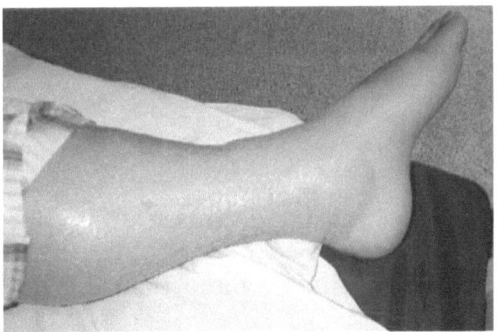

Urinary Symptoms

- Excessive urination at night.
- Frothy urine – May be a sign of protein loss.
- Colour – Colour of urine indicates overall hydration. In kidney dysfunction or jaundice, the urine will be highly coloured.
- Pain and burning sensation during urination – It indicates infection of the urinary tract. Fever along with these symptoms is more suggestive of infection.

Blood in urine

There can be frank blood in urine or urine mixed with blood. This can occur in various diseases.

- Kidney stones
- Urinary tract infection

- Kidney Cancer
- Nephritis

Decreased urine output

Daily urine output of less than 500 ml consistently is a sign of kidney failure. Accurate measurement and quantification of urine are a must in disease states.

Excessive urination is due to multiple causes

- Coffee and other beverages
- Alcohol
- Diabetes mellitus
- Kidney dysfunction
- Hormonal imbalance causing decreased urine concentration

Unusually excessive urine of more than 3.5 litres in adults also needs to be evaluated.

Other symptoms of kidney diseases

- High Blood Pressure
- Loss of appetite
- Vomiting
- Back pain
- Itching
- Difficulty in breathing

Must remember – Kidney disease without symptoms

In most instances, kidney disease can progress without any symptoms. Therefore, periodic health check-ups, especially after 40 years and in those with a family history of kidney disease play a pivotal role in the identification of these diseases.

Common Investigations in Kidney Diseases

Creatinine

It is a chemical that is released from the muscles into the bloodstream continuously. Kidneys eliminate them through urinary excretion. In the event of kidney dysfunction, the levels of creatinine increase in the blood which is easily quantifiable.

Apart from creatinine, various other biochemical products accumulate in the event of kidney failure which is not easily measurable and not routinely done.

Urea

Like creatinine, it is another metabolic end product that accumulates in the event of kidney failure.

GFR – Glomerular Filtration Rate

It is a very important and accurate measure of kidney function than creatinine itself. It is calculated from a formula that involves creatinine level, age, sex and weight. With the same level of creatinine, GFR will vary with various age groups and physique.

Other blood tests

- Hemoglobin
- Sodium/potassium/phosphorus/uric acid/albumin
- Blood sugar
- Blood cholesterol

Urine test

- Very easy and inexpensive
- A small quantity of urine is enough
- Early morning urine sampling is ideal
- We can evaluate for protein in the urine

- Evidence for infection can be sought

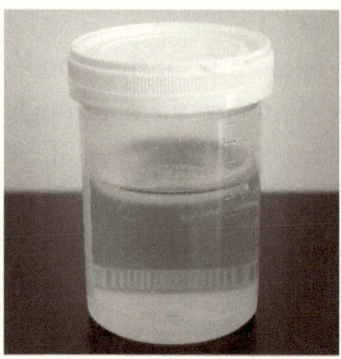

For accurate quantification of proteinuria
- Microalbuminuria
- 24-hour urine protein – Urine sample should be collected over a whole day and protein excretion should be calculated

Ultrasound Scan

The dimensions of the kidneys can be assessed using ultrasound. It is useful for the identification of kidney cysts and stones.

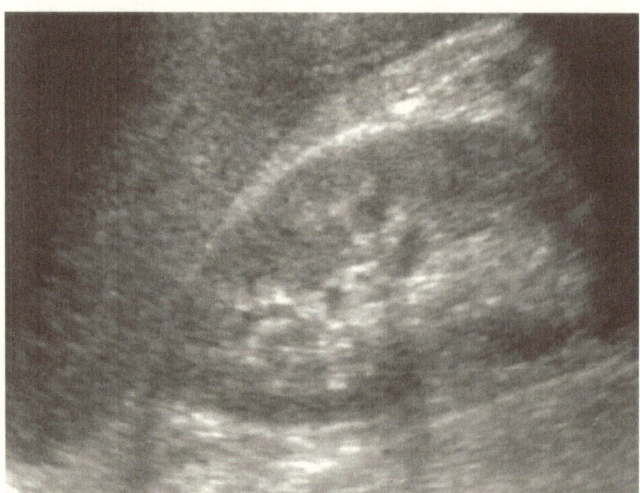

CT scan

Swelling of the kidney, kidney infection, kidney stones and obstruction can be accurately assessed using a computerised tomogram (CT Scan)

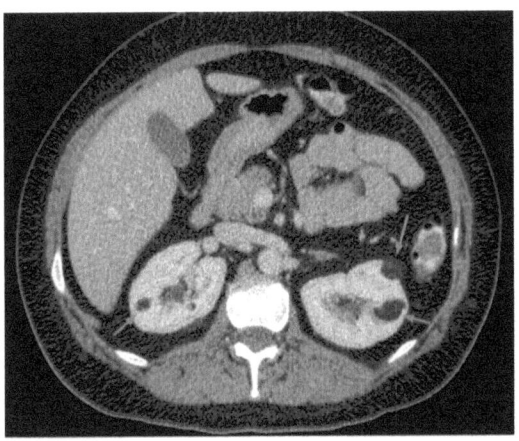

Kidney tissue testing (Kidney biopsy)

A kidney biopsy is essential for accurate diagnosis of kidney disease and in instances when the disease could not be diagnosed by other modes. A tissue sample is taken from the kidney, usually under local anaesthesia. The tissue is processed and viewed with a microscope. The doctor will explain the pros and cons before embarking on the test.

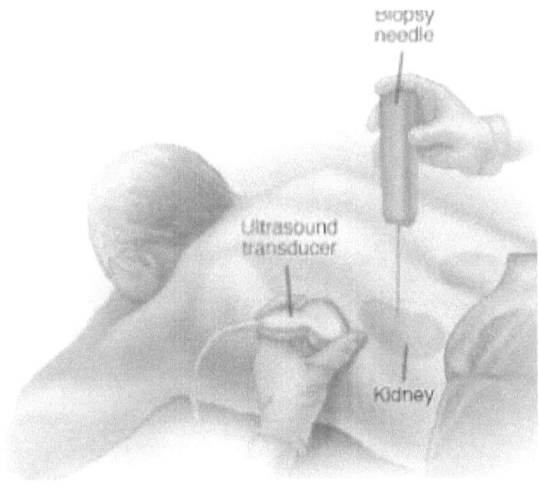

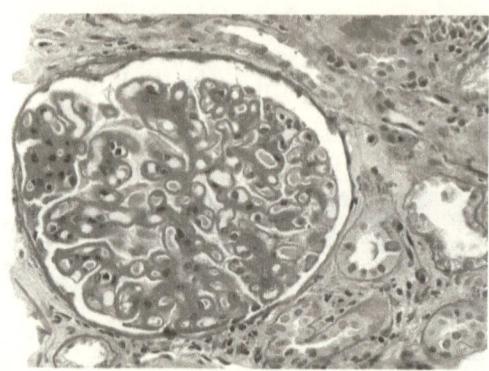

When biopsy (tissue examination) cannot be done?

- Decreased dimensions of the kidney
- Very high creatinine
- Poor blood clotting
- Patient on blood-thinning medications.

Nuclear scan examination

Used for an accurate measure of GFR, obstruction and kidney scars.

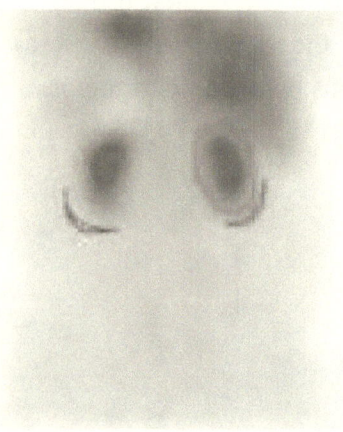

"Diagnosing a kidney disease is simpler than the disease of most other organs."

Kidney Disease – The Real Problem

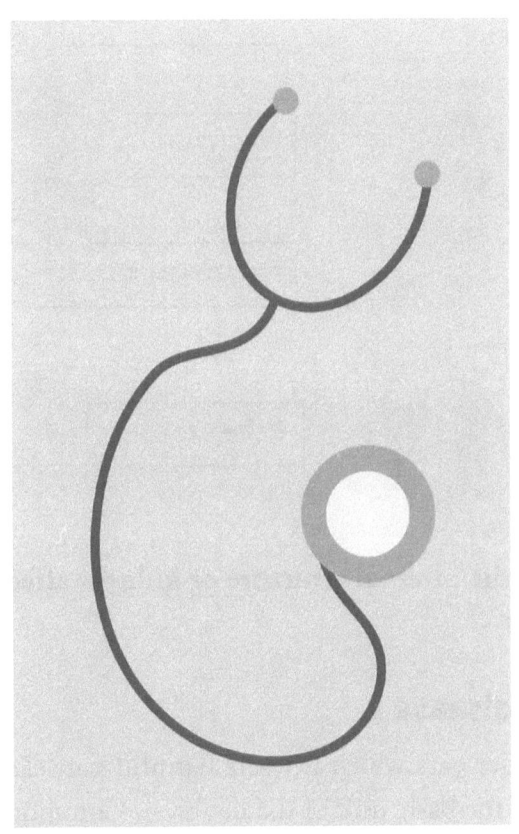

Kidney failure – Causal factors

For every ten people afflicted by chronic kidney failure, the probable causes are enlisted below.

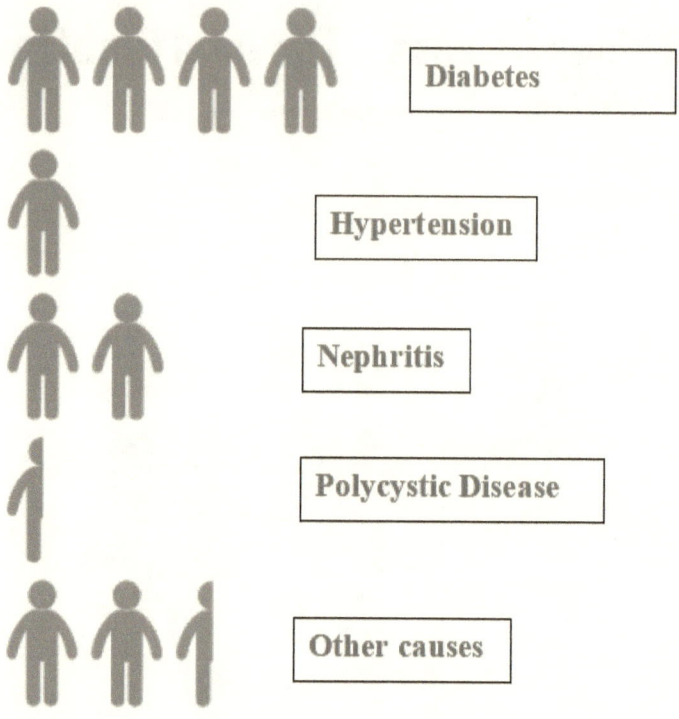

Basic facts on the internal structure of kidneys affected by various kidney diseases

Glomerular disease

In the kidney, the part which extracts harmful particles from blood is the glomerulus, the basic unit of the nephron. Common causes of renal failure such as **diabetes and hypertension** affects this portion of the nephron, causing kidney dysfunction.

Interstitial disease

Infection and toxic drugs affect this part of the kidney, which is the space between each nephron, eventually leads to kidney failure.

Kidney infection

Kidney infections are caused by bacteria and other microorganisms. Women are more prone to kidney infections. Both acute and chronic kidney failure can occur which can be prevented by early identification of the symptoms.

Renal blood vessel obstruction

High cholesterol and smoking can affect kidney blood vessels. This eventually leads to high blood pressure and shrinkage of the kidneys. This is referred to as renal artery stenosis. At times this can lead to a sudden onset of difficulty in breathing requiring emergency medical attention.

Urinary tract obstruction

Enlargement of the prostate gland in men and cervical cancer in women are common causes of urinary tract obstruction which eventually leads to renal failure if left untreated.

Kidney cyst (Polycystic disease)

These are genetic diseases. Hundreds of cysts (swelling with liquid content) form in the kidneys gradually. This leads to hypertension and kidney damage but nevertheless is preventable.

Kidney stones

Kidney stones can be found in any part of the urinary tract including the kidneys, ureter or urinary bladder.

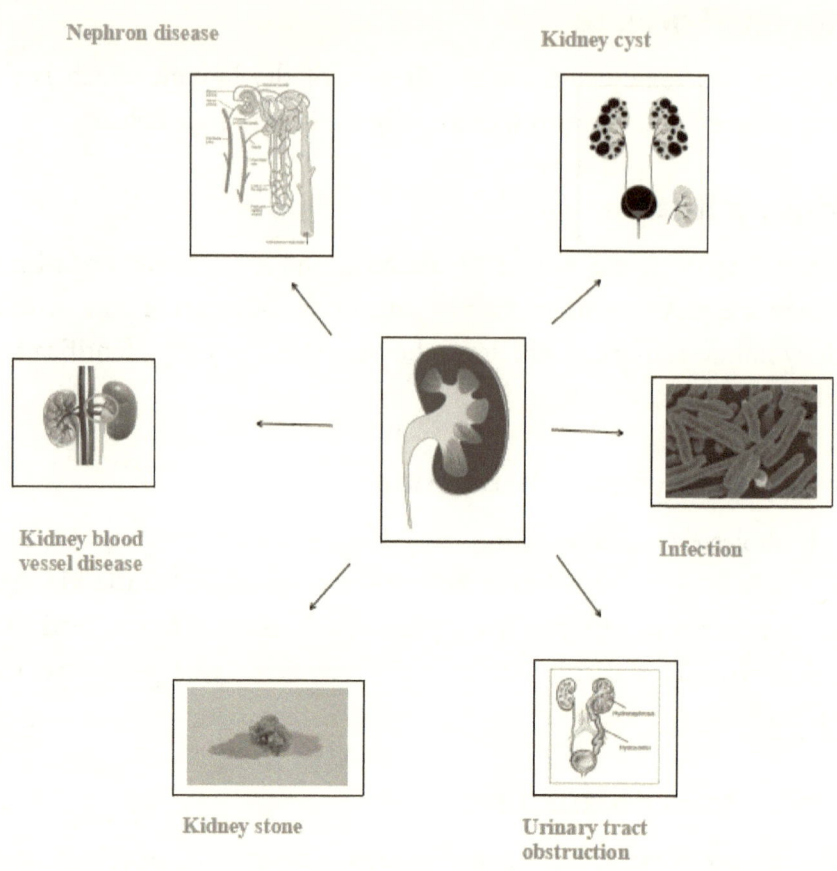

The major group of kidney diseases

"There are a few groups of kidney diseases which culminate in kidney failure if not cared for."

Sugar Bites – Kidney Disease in Diabetes

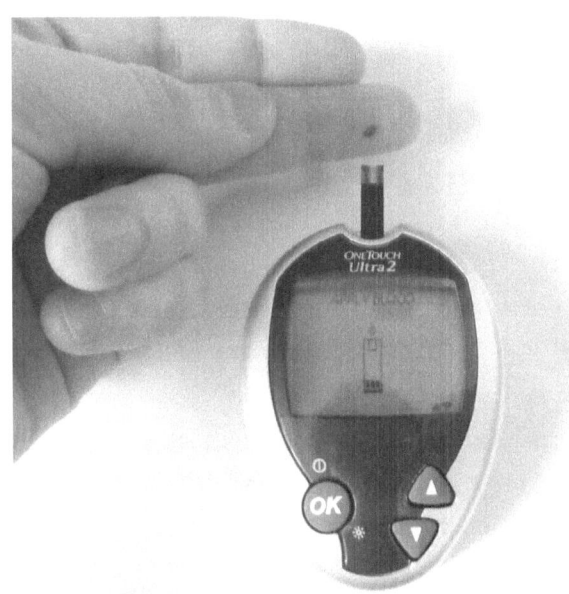

"Diabetes sounds like you're going to die when you hear it. I was immediately frightened. But once I got a better idea of what it was and that it was something, I could manage myself, I was comforted."

– Nick Jonas (American actor & Singer)

I should narrate the story of one of my patient whose blood sugar level rose to soaring levels.

Mr. Raj was in his mid-fifties and a diabetic for more than 10 years. He has a fairly good knowledge of his diabetes status and gets consultation on a bi-monthly basis. But the sugars were always on the higher side. His last visit with his diabetologist was around 40 days back.

He came to the emergency department with chest pain. He was otherwise well preserved. Initial lab tests were sent and medicines for his heart were pumped in. The result came and his blood sugar was whooping 1250 mg/dl (69.57 mmol/l.) This is more than 10 times the normal value. He was sitting and talking though.

I knew that the highest blood sugar recorded in a survivor was with Michael Patrick Buonocore (USA) and he survived a blood sugar level of 147.6 mmol/L (2,656 mg/dl.) He found a place for himself in the Guinness book of world records.

We have also seen values nearing 1500 mg/dl but usually, those were sick and fatal most of the time. For our patient, we started on a drip of insulin and he came out of it well.

The last time when he had his sugars checked, also had a check of urine. His urine protein showed 4+ and his kidneys were under-functioning. These patients with chronically high blood sugars suffer organ damage, which in most situations are not completely reversible.

Beware of the heart, kidney, brain and eyes if you have diabetes.

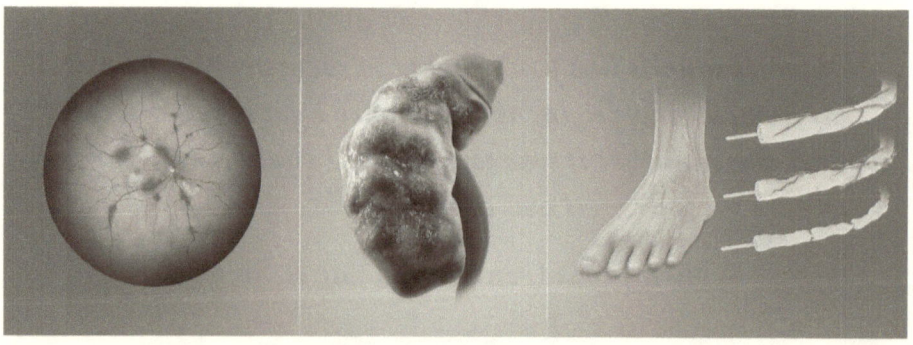

Regarding Diabetes
What causes it?
Diabetes occurs due to decreased secretion of insulin or the inability of the secreted insulin to act properly. This causes increased sugar levels in the blood and consequently diabetes.

Type 1:
It occurs at a young age due to viral infection or an unknown factor causing damage to the insulin-secreting pancreas. It loses the capacity to secrete insulin. Taking insulin injections is mandatory in this group of patients.

Type 2:
Generally occurs after thirty years of age. It is due to genetic factors and lifestyle changes. Initially, it gets controlled with drugs but later during the course of the disease one may require insulin.

Why does diabetes-related kidney disease occur?
Persistent high blood sugars cause harmful end products that damage the kidneys. The minute blood vessels in the kidneys gets damaged. Keeping the blood sugar in check is the ideal way to protect the kidneys from the harmful effects of diabetes.

Who has more chance to get diabetes-related kidney disease?
- 30 to 40% of diabetic patients have a chance to get a kidney ailment
- Long-term diabetics
- Persons with uncontrolled blood sugar
- Persons with persistent high blood pressure
- Obesity
- Smoking
- Usually, diabetic kidney disease occurs in conjunction with diabetes-related nerve damage (neuropathy) and retina damage (retinopathy)

Timeline of Onset of Kidney Damage Due to Diabetes

TYPE-I Diabetes Patients:

At least ten years from the onset of diabetes.

TYPE-II Diabetes Patients:

Cannot be determined. Can occur any time after the diagnosis.

How does kidney damage begin and progress?

For most patients, excessive urine protein (albumin) excretion will be the initial stage of kidney damage due to diabetes. If left unattended it may progress to renal dysfunction. Importantly all these may progress without any symptoms and the only way of detection is regular follow-up. Blood sugar levels may decrease as kidney dysfunction progresses.

How to prevent diabetes-related kidney damage?
- Detect diabetes early
- Blood pressure to be maintained less than 140/90 mm Hg at all times
- Urine protein to be tested at least once a year
- Take less salt
- Control weight gain and increase physical activity
- If your family member has diabetes-related kidney disease you should be very careful
- Newer drugs – Some newer drugs prevent and delay the onset of diabetes-related kidney disease

What should be done after the onset of diabetes-related kidney disease?
- Dietary modifications
- Try to reduce protein excretion in urine with the help of drugs
- Regular follow-up of creatinine level in the blood

- Studies have shown that improving long-term blood glucose control can greatly reduce the risk of progressive kidney damage.

What are other common kidney problems which can occur in diabetes?
- Urinary tract infection/Pyelonephritis (Infection of the kidneys)
- Shrinkage of blood vessels of the kidney (Renal Artery Stenosis)
- Kidney stones

Is it completely possible to prevent kidney damage if you are having long-standing diabetes?
Yes, very much possible

Former Pakistan cricket all-rounder Wasim Akram was diagnosed with diabetes at the age of thirty. He had to take insulin daily. He created major records only after the onset of diabetes. Even now at the age of fifty, after about 20 years of diagnosis he is fit and roaring!

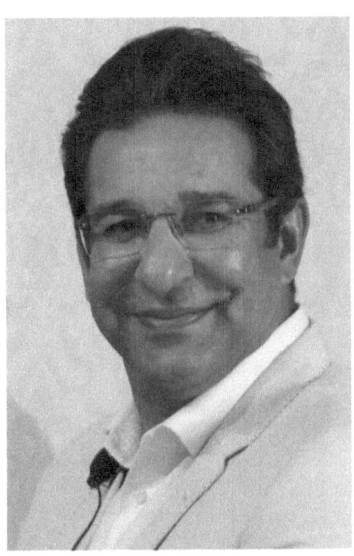

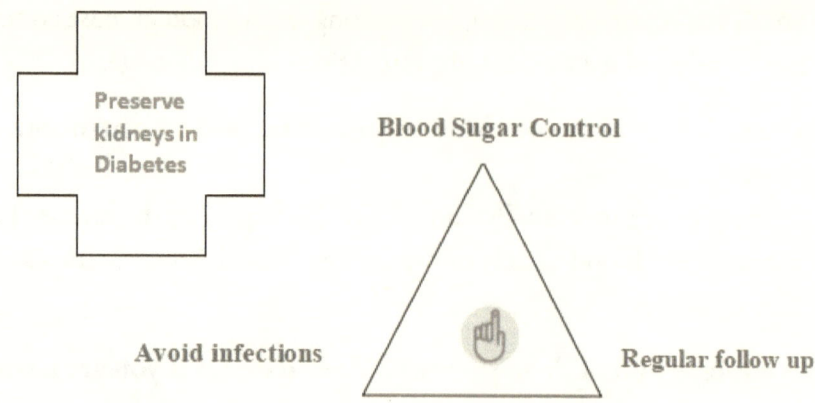

> *"People think it's hard to cut out sugar, but it can be done. You just have to put some effort in."*
>
> – Halle Berry, Hollywood Actor

It is estimated that 4 out of every 10 people with diabetes develop nephropathy at some point during their illness. Diabetes control gives immense benefits and protects every cell and organ from progressive damage.

Blood Pressure and the Kidneys

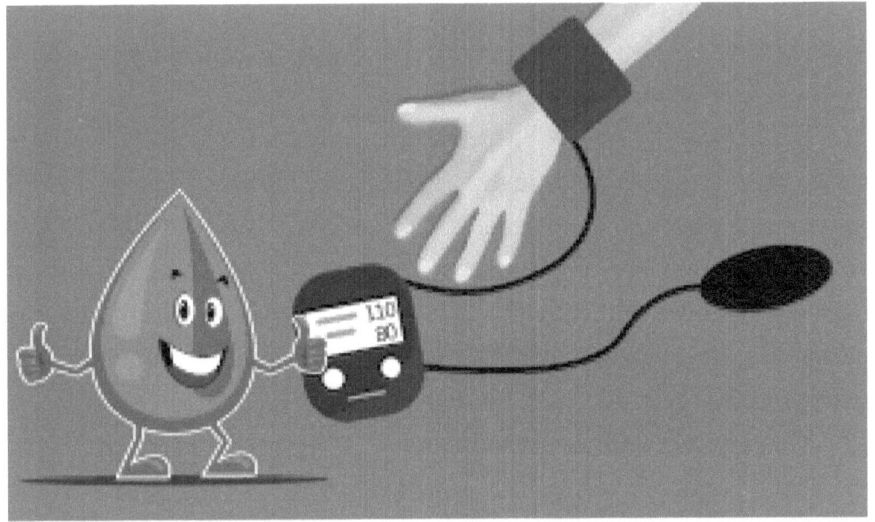

"If you don't know your blood pressure, it's like not knowing the value of your company."

– Mehmet Oz

"280/160 mm Hg"

My staff nurse uttered to me when I asked to check the blood pressure of an elderly gentleman we received in the emergency room at the end of that day.

It is the pressure that blood exerts on the blood tubes all over the body from head to foot.

The delicate blood vessels of the kidney bear the brunt of the attack. Rupture of blood vessels can make his brain to be filled with blood clots and make him unconscious and the kidneys may stop filtering blood to remove the toxins or make urine.

He was having slightly higher blood pressure and his kidney has been working below normal over the past few months and was on follow up in another hospital in the city.

We have to lower the blood pressure significantly within minutes or face the consequences. Luckily right now he is talking well and he has only muscle pain and no serious symptoms.

We started on blood pressure lowering medications through intravenous route and sent the necessary tests. His already hampered kidney function had got a further hit due to high blood pressure. Yes, he was on the verge of requiring dialysis.

We gave multiple drugs to control his hypertension except for the one which is not given in severe renal failure.

The next day the blood pressure was ravaging around 250 mm Hg. The blood test that came over the next day revealed that he had a rare disease called Scleroderma. It usually affects other organs and skin changes do occur. He didn't have any skin problems though. The drug which was held as he had severe renal failure should now be given to him as a treatment for this disease.

His blood pressure then started to trend down. Kidneys began to recover slowly and we avoided dialysis.

It was a great sigh of relief for the patient and the family.

Beware High Blood Pressure Can Strike in Any Form
Analysis of research

High blood pressure is a widely prevalent disease. Its impact is felt more in the urban areas than in the rural and village zones. There is not a single symptom that specifically denotes hypertension. Aptly it is called the silent killer. Only early detection and prevention of this killer disease will prevent further organ damage.

What is high blood pressure?

The blood pumped out from the heart exerts pressure on all the blood vessels of the body. If the exerted pressure becomes high it affects both larger and smaller blood vessels of the body. Uncontrolled blood pressure affects multiple organs in the body.

There are two measurements in blood pressure?
Upper: Systolic – 90 to 140 mm Hg
Lower: Diastolic – 60 to 90 mm Hg
Most denotes this average as 120/80 mm Hg of blood pressure.

Two types

High blood pressure can be of two types
1. Primary Hypertension
2. Secondary Hypertension

Primary hypertension

The cause of high blood pressure is related to factors in the kidney and high salt intake. There will be no identifiable cause for this blood pressure. It affects people around 30 to 50 years of age.

This is the commonest form of hypertension across the world. If one has a parent or a family member affected by high blood pressure, he or she has a high chance to get the disease if adequate lifestyle changes are not instituted.

Secondary hypertension

A rare form of high blood pressure occurring in 5-15 % of hypertensives and most of the time blood pressure is uncontrollable. There is more chance of organ damage in this group of patients.

Causes
- Kidney failure
- Renal artery stenosis
- Changes in adrenal and thyroid glands
- Some drugs
- Heart valve defects

Can blood pressure be inherited (genetic)?
Blood pressure is probably a multifactorial disease. Genetic influence can be a factor but is not the sole cause. For the same reason, lifestyle changes can prevent or control high blood pressure.

What impacts will there be?
Uncontrolled high blood pressure affects most organs in the body. Around 10% to 20% of hypertensives develop kidney disease at some point in time.

Hypertension – Affected Organs

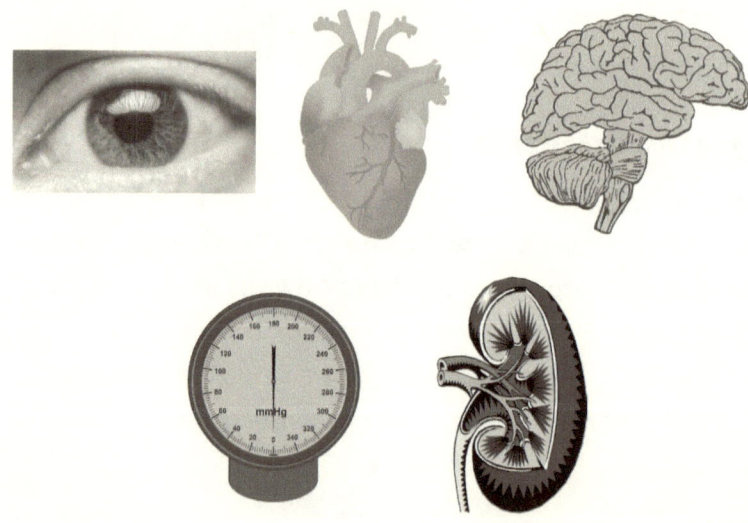

Salt and blood pressure

When the amount of salt is high in the diet it has to be eliminated by the kidneys. Then only the salt balance is maintained in the body. Once excessive salt is taken, it can be pushed out only by increasing the blood pressure. The excessive salt is thus excreted and the balance is achieved.

If the salt intake is high over a period of time, the high blood pressure sustains. This also affects the quality of the blood vessels, making them stiffer. The blood pressure is then persistently elevated. Then we need drugs to lower the blood pressure.

Salt and kidney – Effects

- High blood Pressure
- High urine protein excretion
- Kidney Stone
- Reduces kidney function directly

How is high blood pressure identified?

In most instances, there will not be any symptoms. Occasionally there may be giddiness and headache. Blood pressure measurement should be done periodically after 30 years of age.

Diagnosis

Physicians may take two or three readings before diagnosing hypertension.

What tests will be carried out?

- Urine & Blood investigations
- ECG
- Echocardiogram
- Eye examination
- Blood vessels screening (Doppler study)
- Ultrasound Abdomen to assess the kidneys

Ambulatory blood pressure monitoring

Most often the blood pressure taken in the doctor's room may be variably high or low. A blood pressure machine is put on your arm and it records the blood pressure over a 24 hours period. This mode is very useful in assessing the trend of blood pressure and choosing the right type of drugs.

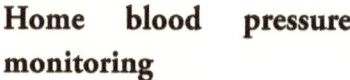

Home blood pressure monitoring

- A simple measure to track blood pressure periodically.
- Reassures the control of blood pressure and motivates for continued medication intake.
- If home blood pressure is high one should enquire with the doctor regarding alteration of medications.

Medications for blood pressure – Things to note

1. The drugs prescribed to you for hypertension depends on the blood pressure reading and your other health conditions.
2. More than one drug may be needed at times.
3. If a particular drug is intolerant or not working for you, should approach the doctor for alternative drugs. Simply stopping the drug will lead to complications.
4. When there is an occurrence of dehydration (vomiting, diarrhoea, blood loss) one should stop the drugs and approach the doctor.

"High blood pressure is the real silent enemy.
It takes less than a minute to know your blood pressure control."

Kidney Stones

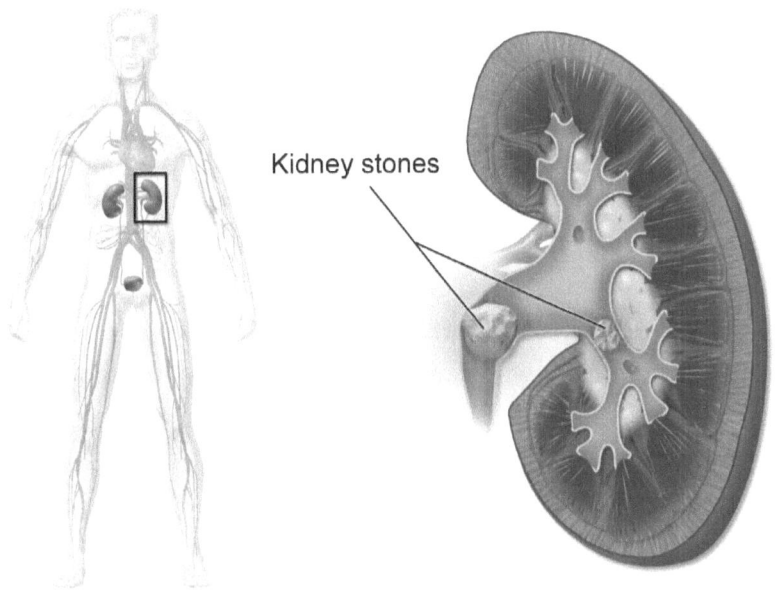

"I aimed at moving mountains, Then Kidney Stone happened to me and now I couldn't take a few steps.."

– Nilofer Kapadia

At five o'clock in the morning, my phone bell rang.

"Hello!"

My family friend was on the other end.

"My brother has severe abdomen pain and vomiting since last night."

"Okay, come straight to the hospital."

I went rushing to the hospital immediately.

On enquiry patient uttered,

"Doctor! There was a similar problem a year ago. You did a scan and said there was a stone in one of the kidneys. In a few days, the stone came out spontaneously. When you were informed over the phone, you told me to come for review and follow up investigations. But we never turned up after that incident."

At forty-five, he was found to be obese.

He was promptly administered with medications to reduce pain. One of the first things you are taught after medical school is how to diagnose and manage renal colic (pain of a kidney stone). It is very rewarding to see the patient calming down after a single intramuscular injection who was previously wincing and shouting with extreme pain. In the case of recurrent stones, most patients diagnose themselves with the occurrence of characteristic symptoms like pain and vomiting.

His painful episode got better over the next fifteen minutes. We immediately proceeded with a simple ultrasound scan of the urinary system. There were two stones in the right kidney and two in the left kidney.

I sat down in my chamber along with my friend and his family members to discuss further courses as for any other patient. I tried to explain in detail.

"This is a mistake many of us make. We don't follow measures to prevent stone formation. Even after the diagnosis of stone for the first time, we are reluctant. We don't take the necessary steps for prevention and hence suffer from recurrent stone formation. Studies have shown that, once kidney

stone has formed, over five years period there is a fifty percent chance of new stone formation."

The patient felt guilty for not following up with the doctor regularly.

"Well, doctor! We will adhere to your instructions from now on."

Why do we get the stones?
Every year, thousands of patients suffer from kidney stones and seek emergency treatment. Lifestyle changes are a major cause of the currently increasing number of patients with kidney stones.

What are kidney stones?
Kidney stones are large concretions formed from chemical substances in the urine. Normally other than toxic substances, salts, minerals and chemicals are excreted in the urine. Decreased solubility or increased concentration of certain substances in urine make them slowly deposit in the urinary tract. They start as small stones and slowly increase in size.

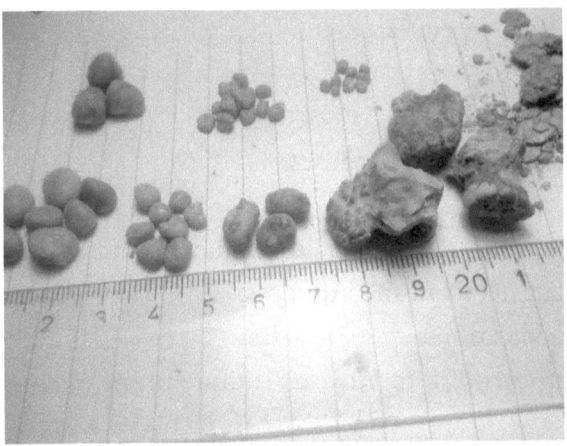

What happens to the stones?
The kidney stone may stay in the kidneys or move slowly and reach the urinary tube (ureter) or the urinary bladder. Occasionally stones can form in the urinary bladder also.

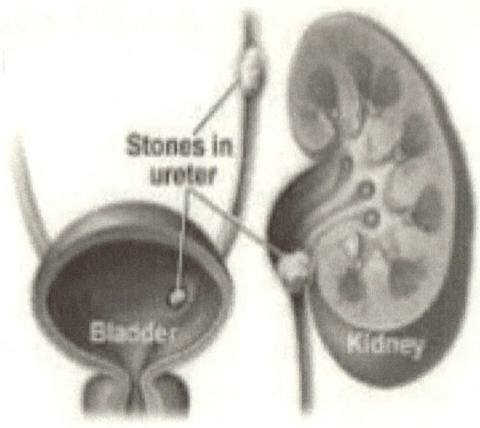

Size

It can be barely visible to as large as the size of a cricket ball. Some stones of staghorn type will occupy almost whole of the kidney.

What is the risk that one forms a stone?
- Less water intake
- Obesity
- Excessive non-vegetarian diet
- Alcoholism
- Kidney infection
- Hereditary diseases (rare causes)
- Diabetes mellitus
- Excessive excretion of uric acid/calcium/oxalic acid in urine due to the inherent defect in the kidneys
- Certain medications
- The age group of 20 to 50 years is more prone to stone formation

Does stress aggravate stone formation?
The latest research has shown that stress causes hormonal changes. This leads to decreased solubility of chemicals in urine and leads to the formation of stones.

What are the symptoms of urinary tract stones?
- Most kidney stones are free of any symptoms. They cause symptoms when they increase in size or block any part of the urinary tract.
- Pain in the lower back, radiating to the abdomen or thigh sometimes associated with vomiting.
- Frequent urination
- Urine mixed with blood
- Sometimes stones come out during urination
- May cause urinary tract infections
- Urinary tract stones (ureter) will cause more symptoms than kidney stones

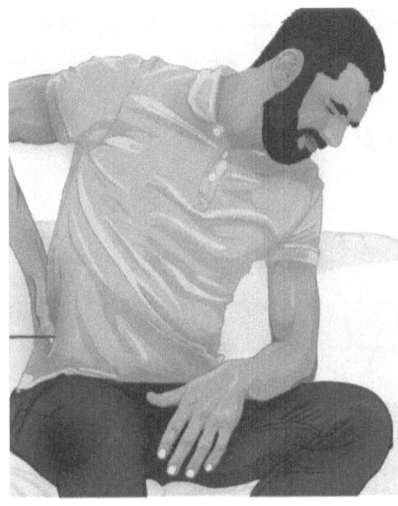

Do Stones cause Kidney failure?
If symptoms are unattended, it can also cause kidney failure.

Initial Tests
Urine Test
To find out if there is an associated infection, sometimes it can give a clue to the type of stone.

Kidney function tests:

Urea and creatinine in the blood.

Scan:

Ultrasound or CT scan can accurately determine the size of the stone and its location.

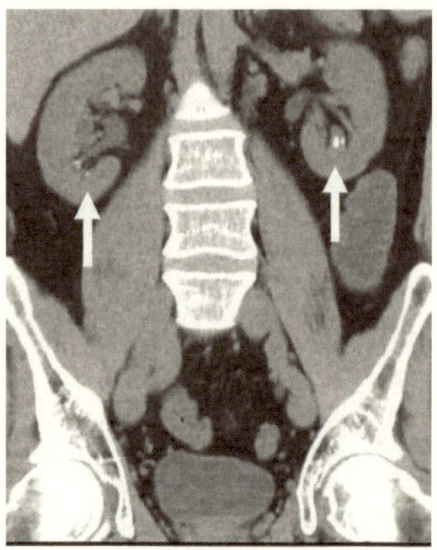

Types of kidney stones

- Calcium oxalate (over 75%)
- Calcium phosphate
- Struvite stones
- Uric acid stones

What to do next?

Smaller stones are more likely to pass in urine spontaneously. Only pain relief is needed. Stones causing obstruction causes enlargement of the kidneys. Long-standing obstruction leads to loss of kidney function. These types of stones may need to be removed quickly. Surgical procedures vary depending upon the location and size of the stones.

Methods of removal of stones:
- Endoscopic removal – Ureteroscopy (URS) and Retrograde intrarenal surgery (RIRS)
- Extracorporeal shockwave lithotripsy (ESWL)
- Surgical procedures (Percutaneous or open)

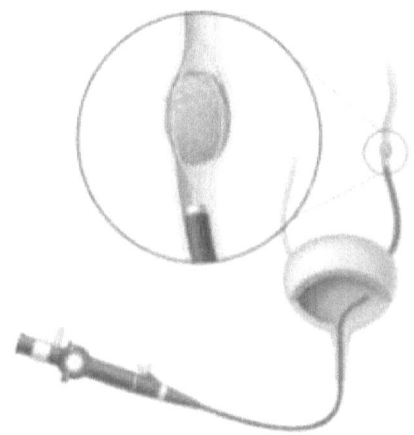

Second-line investigations

They are useful in preventing recurrent stone formation.

Urine is collected over 24 hours and its chemical composition will be analysed.

- Calcium
- Phosphorus
- Uric Acid
- Oxalic acid
- Citric acid

Kidney stone analysis

Stones removed during surgical procedures will be subjected to analysis of their composition.

Based on the reports exact dietary modification will be done.

Are there any medications available to treat stones?
Magnesium and citric acid prevent the formation of stones. Most stone prevention medicines contain these supplements

Can I resort to alternative medicine?
Make sure that any medication you take is certified and approved.

What are the situations requiring urgent treatment for kidney stones?
- High-grade fever
- Persistent and severe pain
- People with kidney failure
- Uncontrolled diabetes
- Urine retention within kidneys

Other dietary measures to reduce the occurrence of kidney stones are enumerated in chapter 27.

> *"The best method to treat kidney stones is to prevent them from getting formed."*

How Germs Attack the Kidneys?

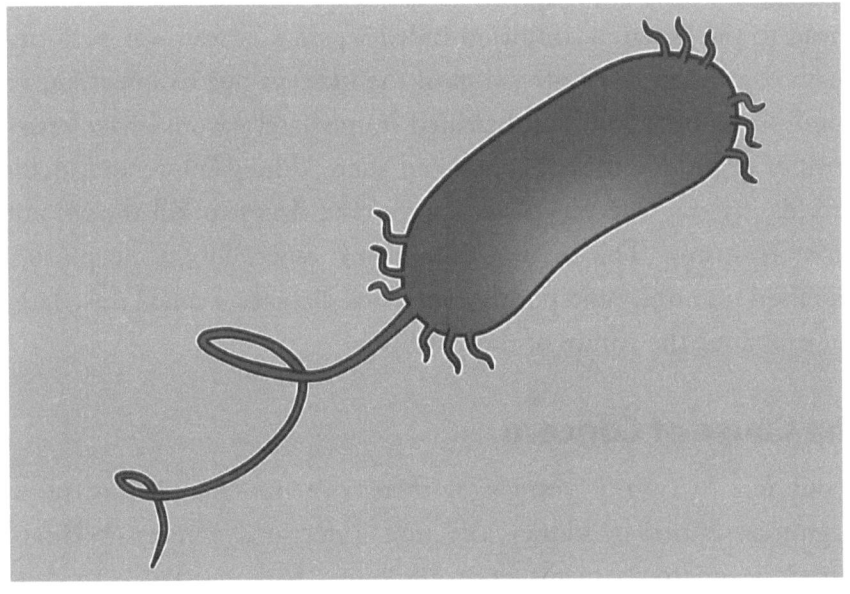

*"If human numbers increase the rate
of infection also increases."*

– William H. McNeill (Plague and People)

At the intensive care unit, a patient was recuperating well.

The incidents which unfolded a week earlier flashed through my mind.

I encountered an elderly female in the emergency ward.

She was brought to our hospital in a gasping state, referred from a hospital in the nearby town. Her body was cold and clammy. Her pulse was barely felt and the blood pressure was also not recordable. On inquiry, she was suffering from fever for a week. She had back pain and also uncontrolled blood sugar levels.

She was immediately put on an artificial respirator.

She had urinary tract infection. Infection of the kidneys had spread to the blood, a condition called sepsis. CT scan was performed which confirmed the destruction of the kidneys due to infection. Her blood-borne infection if not treated immediately, would have created a risk of death due to sepsis. She had acute kidney failure and inching towards dialysis. She was given appropriate drugs to kill the invading microorganisms. This is not infrequent especially in people with depressed immunity and poorly controlled diabetes. I called the relatives and explained the nature of the condition.

The Cause of Concern

About ten to twenty years ago, there was no renal failure of this magnitude caused by kidney infection. Infections were easily curable. Currently, microorganisms have developed high resistance to drugs. Microorganisms don't succumb even to the powerful drugs. When these infections are overwhelmed, it is more likely to cause permanent kidney failure. Early detection of symptoms not only prevents renal failure but also saves cost and life.

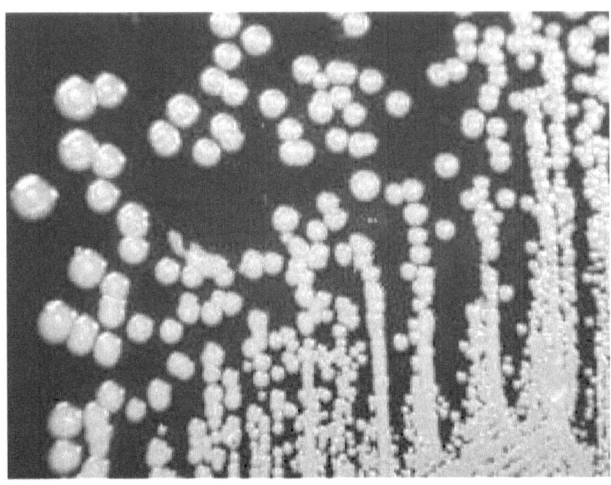

Symptoms of urinary tract infection

- Irritation during or after urination
- Pain over back & lower abdomen
- Fever with chills
- Vomiting
- Blood in urine
- Frequent urination

The above symptoms may be present alone or in combination.

Complicated urinary tract infection

This group of patients should be extremely careful as they can suffer more damage if the infection is not treated early and adequately.

1. Infection in pregnancy
2. Urinary tract anomalies
3. Urinary catheters
4. Those who have undergone a kidney transplant
5. People with diabetes
6. Those with depressed immunity (Cancer, HIV, organ transplant)
7. Presence of stones in the urinary tract

These patients often require inpatient treatment.

Pyelonephritis
- It is the infection of the kidney tissue
- One or both kidneys may be affected
- Can lead to acute kidney failure
- Early aggressive treatment is necessary

Tests required in patients with urinary tract infection?
- Urine complete evaluation and urine culture
- Blood investigations to identify the complications
- Ultrasound Scan
- CT scan (to be decided on a case to case basis)

Treatment duration

The duration of medications can vary from 5 days to 4 weeks depending on the nature of the infection. Similarly, the need for a pill or injection may vary depending on the severity of the infection.

How to prevent it?
- Drink plenty of water (3-4 liters per day).
- Avoid holding urine for a long time(more than 3 hours).
- Urinate after intercourse.
- It is better to wear cotton inner-wear.
- If you get an infection, complete the full course of the given antibiotics.
- If there is a frequent infection, one may require long-term antibiotics.
- Bacteria can be transmitted to the kidney from the reproductive organs or gastrointestinal tract. Women who are frequently infected should undergo a gynecologist consultation.

> *"Urinary tract infection will most often have an underlying trigger. Identify them early."*

Protein Loss in Urine and Remedies

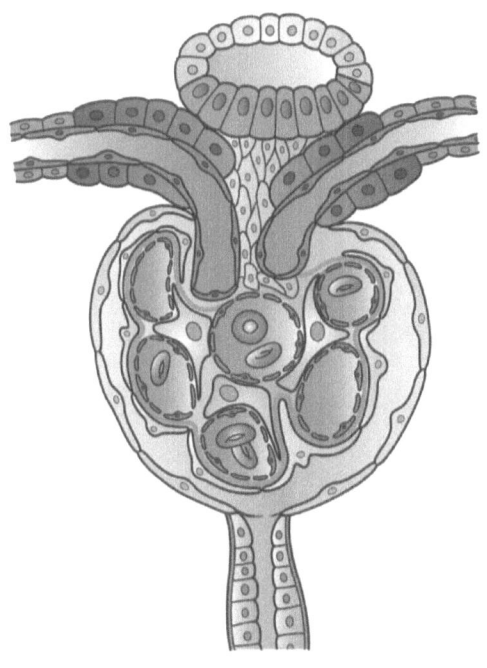

Dharini was the first patient I happened to see on that day, a child around four years of age. The child's mother was nervous. The girl's face and legs were swollen. The child had nephrotic syndrome. I counseled her mother.

"This is a condition that occurs in children. Protein is excreted in the urine, resulting in water clogging between the tissues as edema of the feet and swollen face."

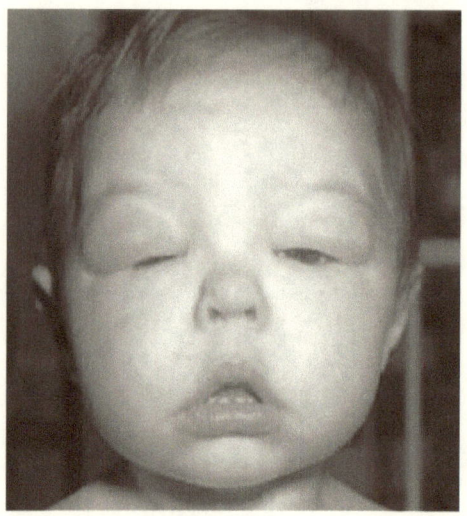

What causes it?
Nephrons are the basic filtering unit of the kidneys. When these nephrons are inflamed in disease states, the kidney starts leaking protein.

Can the problem occur at any age, Doctor?
It is more common in children less than ten years, for whom it can be easily controlled by medications. But the disease can occur at any age. The causes vary with age.

How will be the kidney function in nephrotic syndrome?
Usually, kidney function is not affected in these groups of patients. Sometimes they may have mild dysfunction.

What other tests should the doctor take?
Other than urine and blood tests, some may also require a kidney biopsy. Most children do not need biopsy. This test may be necessary if the disease is not controlled by the usual drugs.

I saw the blood and urine test reports. I started writing prescriptions.

"Steroids are the essential drugs for this problem along with other supportive drugs."

Doctor, I have heard that steroid medications affect even the health of adults. Will my child have those side effects? I am afraid, doctor.

Yes! Steroid drugs can have side effects. But it is necessary to use them judiciously according to the nature of the kidney disease. After a few weeks, the medication dose will be reduced. The first course is usually for 4 to 16 weeks.

Nephrotic Syndrome – Queries

What are the other supportive measures for nephrotic syndrome?
Supportive medicines to decrease the swelling, prevent infection and blood clotting.

What if steroid medication doesn't work?
Rarely other medications may be needed if steroids don't work well.

Can we monitor the disease at home?
Protein levels in urine can be tested at home using the urine dipstick test.

What diet should we follow?
Salt restriction is a must to get rid of the excessive fluids faster. Protein should be consumed in adequate quantity.

Doctor, will there be any other problems?
Steroids are effective in children. The majority of them respond very well. Some children may need other medications. But don't worry about anything, give medicines regularly with confidence.

I sent them back saying she will recover soon.

Nephrotic syndrome in adults
Reasons:
1. Primary glomerular disease
2. Diabetes mellitus
3. Secondary to Cancer
4. Lupus disease – mainly in women

Medicines in adults vary according to the nature of kidney disease.

Kidney Cysts

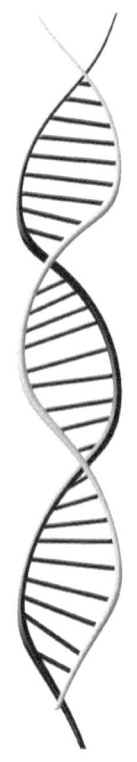

In the critical care unit, I was asked to see a female patient of around 50 years of age. She was admitted with a ruptured swollen blood vessel called an aneurysm, a devastating emergency. It caused the blood to fill all around the brain and its coverings. The aneurysm was just identified and metallic coiling was done to arrest the bleeding. Our radiologist asked me to see her as she had numerous fluid-filled swelling in both her kidneys.

On enquiry, she revealed that her father had also suffered from kidney disease. She was previously well and did not have symptoms. Now her blood pressure was very high requiring intravenous drugs. A scan revealed both her kidneys containing innumerable cysts. She had autosomal dominant polycystic kidney disease. The aneurysm in the brain was possibly due to the same defect as in the kidneys.

Her both kidneys were functioning well at that point in time. Careful follow-up and drugs are required to prevent the growth of the kidney cysts and preserve kidney function.

Polycystic Kidney Disease?

It is a genetic disease. It occurs in two variants, the most common dominant disease is usually diagnosed in adults.

Autosomal Dominant Polycystic Kidney Disease (ADPKD) in Adults

This disease is prevalent in more than 20 million people around the world. The disease causes symptoms at any age group between 30 and 70 years and usually one of the parent or siblings has the same disease. In approximately 15% of cases, ADPKD occurs in people without a family history of the disease (i.e., family members have been evaluated and have no evidence for PKD.)

There is the formation of thousands of small fluid-filled cysts that gradually expand in size. At times the kidney size is enormously increased. Cysts may also grow in other organs, including the liver, pancreas, thyroid gland and/or spleen.

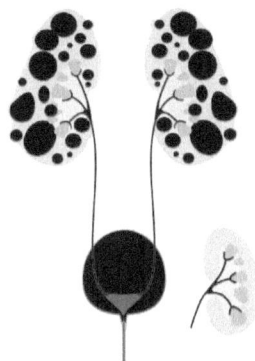

What are the problems faced?
- Enlarged kidneys are most often detected during a health check-up
- High blood pressure
- Abdomen pain and fullness
- Blood in urine
- Kidney stones
- Kidney infection
- Kidney failure
- Cysts in other organs may cause symptoms related to it

What are the tests to be done?
- Kidney scan
- Kidney function tests
- MRI Brain in the presence of neurological symptoms
- Genetic testing

Remedies:
The growth of these cysts is the prime factor for hypertension and renal dysfunction associated with this disease. So suppressing their growth will slow the progression of kidney disease.

Drink a lot of water
Vasopressin is one of the hormones which acts as a growth factor for these cysts. Drinking a lot of water will suppress this hormone and

decrease the growth of the cysts. This will also slow the progression of kidney disease.

Drugs

Drugs to suppress the vasopressin hormone helps to slow the disease process.

Kidney dysfunction

If kidney dysfunction occurs due to the overgrowth of the cysts, it has to be managed accordingly. In the end-stage kidney disease due to ADPKD, fluid intake should be according to the urine output.

Kidney cyst in children (Recessive disease):

The same disease can occur in children but it is rare. The kidneys start to get affected in the mother's womb. Kidney failure is almost inevitable in early childhood.

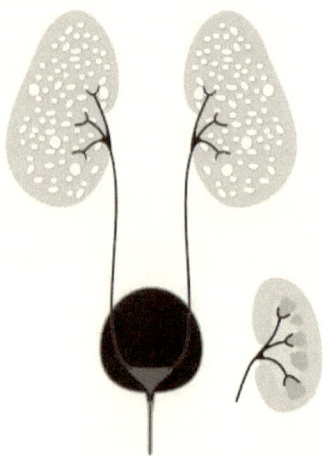

Few other rare diseases also have a genetic role in the transmission.

"Blood pressure control and adequate water intake are the game changers in polycystic kidney disease management."

Kidney Cancer

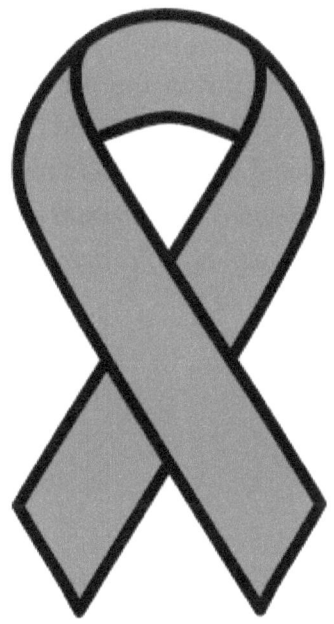

"It's possible not just to survive, but to thrive and to live a healthy, wonderful life again."

– Erika Evans (Cancer survivor)

John was hale and healthy worker in a factory until he noticed a mild high coloured urine a few days back. His body started to show up some unusual signs in the form of not taking the amount of food he used to. He came to me for a consult.

I examined him and ordered a few investigations. His kidney function was normal but his scan showed swelling in the upper part of the left kidney. He didn't have any pain though.

We had a discussion. I knew it was cancer in one of his kidneys. It is an uncontrolled multiplication of the cells of the kidney without any checkpoint. That is how cancer in any part of the body starts and spreads.

Luckily for him, the PET scan and other tests revealed that it has not spread to other parts of the body beyond the kidney.

I discussed this in detail with John and his family members.

Kidney cancer occurs when the normal cells of the kidney change into abnormal cells and grow out of control.

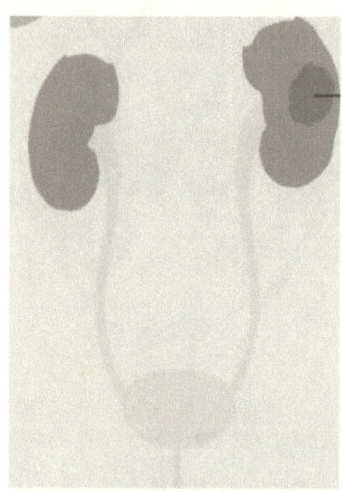

What is the probability that one gets kidney cancer?
In order of occurrence, it is much less common than other cancers such as oral cavity and lungs. The common risks include smoking, hypertension, obesity and occupational exposure to some chemicals.

What are the symptoms?
- Blood in the urine
- Pain on either side of the lower back or over the abdomen
- Weight loss
- Most often detected during a health check-up

What are the tests to confirm the diagnosis?
- USG Abdomen
- CT Scan
- PET scan
- MRI
- Basic blood tests to assess the kidney function

The basis of all the tests is to ascertain whether the cancer is confined to a part or whole kidney and to ascertain its spread elsewhere in the body.

Metastatic cancer is one that can get spread to nearby lymph nodes and other organs or bones.

What is treatment option for kidney cancer?
Surgery
If the cancer is confined to the kidney, removal of cancer along with part or whole of the kidney is curative.

The other kidney takes over the whole function.

Medicines
If the tumour is not operable or has spread to other parts, your doctor will decide on the exact medicines to control the disease.

"Modern medicine can defy the notion – Cancer is incurable."

Kidney Diseases in Children

Few Kidney Diseases Present During Childhood

Congenital Diseases

Due to the changes occurring in the growing foetus in the mother's womb, few congenital diseases can occur. Regular scans during pregnancy can reveal the diseases.

Single Kidney

A child may be born with a single kidney or one kidney may be enlarged and be nonfunctional. It is usually detected during the second trimester anomaly scan.

One kidney is good enough for normal functioning of the body, though one has to take a few precautionary measures.

- Take plenty of water and fluids
- Balanced diet
- Avoid certain pain-relieving medications
- Blood pressure monitoring and control
- Detect stones and infection in early stage
- Avoid engaging in sports that can cause abdominal trauma
- Regular follow up with the Nephrologist.

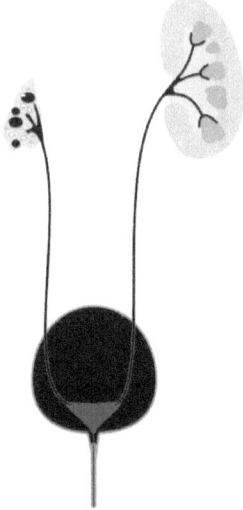

Urinary tract infection in children – Symptoms
- Fever
- Vomiting
- Abdomen pain
- Frequent urination
- Urgency to urinate

Urinary tract infection in children may be due to anatomic abnormality of the kidney or urinary tract. So extensive evaluation is necessary to prevent recurrent infection and future complications.

Other Kidney Problems in Children
Urethral Valve
- Presence of valve at birth in the urinary tract in male children (Posterior urethral valve)
- Defects can be identified in pregnancy scans
- Can cause kidney dysfunction any time since birth
- Endoscopic surgery is curative

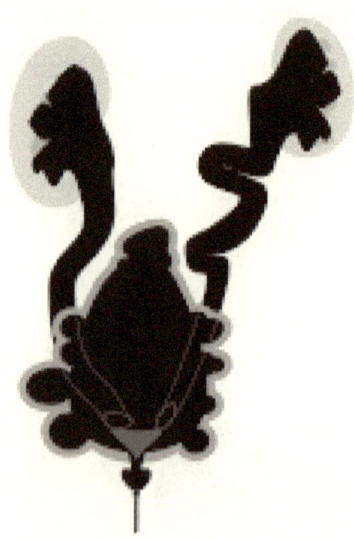

Nephrotic Syndrome/Genetic Diseases

We have discussed this in detail in chapter 9 & 12.

Rickets

Due to defects in the kidneys, calcium and phosphorus balance is affected leading to bony deformity and stunted growth. If the defect is corrected bone growth will be normalised.

Vesico ureteric reflux

Urine refluxes from the urinary bladder to the ureter and kidney due to loss of protective mechanism and defect in the valve.

Problems encountered are

- Frequent urination
- Night time urination
- Urinary tract infections
- Kidney failure
- Child's growth may be affected

Medications or surgical treatment is necessary depending on the severity of the damage

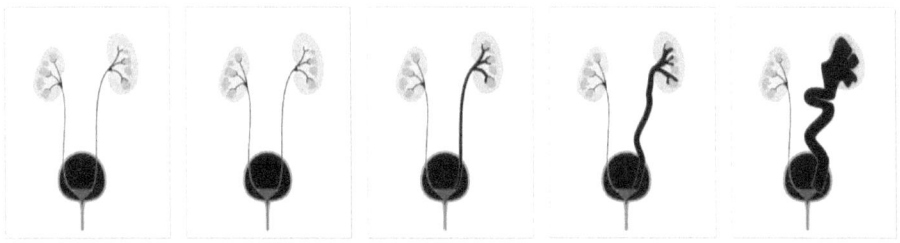

Bed wetting during the night (Nocturnal enuresis)

Bed wetting (also called night time or nocturnal enuresis) is one of the most common childhood problems worrying many parents.

Children usually learn to control daytime urination as they become aware of their bladder filling. This generally occurs within four years of age. Night-time bladder control is attained between 5 and 7 years.

At 10 years, 5% of children continue to bed wet at night time. This is less likely to be due to a major disease.

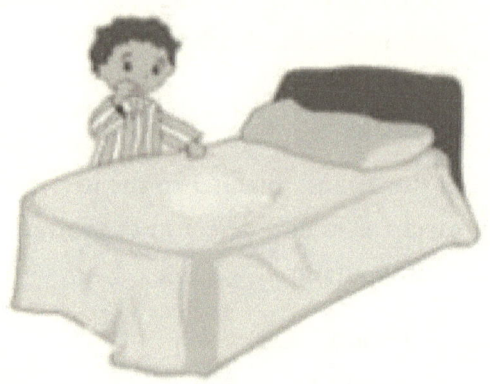

When to approach a physician for bed wetting in the night time?
1. Uncontrolled urination in daytime
2. Increased frequency of urination
3. Worrisome symptoms during urination
4. Extreme tiredness
5. Protein in urine
6. Weight loss
7. Associated Neurological symptoms
8. Symptoms after a period of dry nights
9. Problems with defecation

Remedies
1. Basic investigations
2. Lifestyle measures
3. Drugs if required

Chronic kidney failure in children
It can occur in hereditary diseases and some acquired diseases.

1. There will be a growth retardation
2. Hormonal imbalance
3. Bony deformities
4. Need for kidney supportive medications
5. Dialysis – If kidney failure reaches the end-stage

Blood in urine in children
1. Urinary tract infection
2. Kidney stones
3. Injury
4. Nephritis

"Educate children about the importance of kidney health."

Kidney Diseases in Women

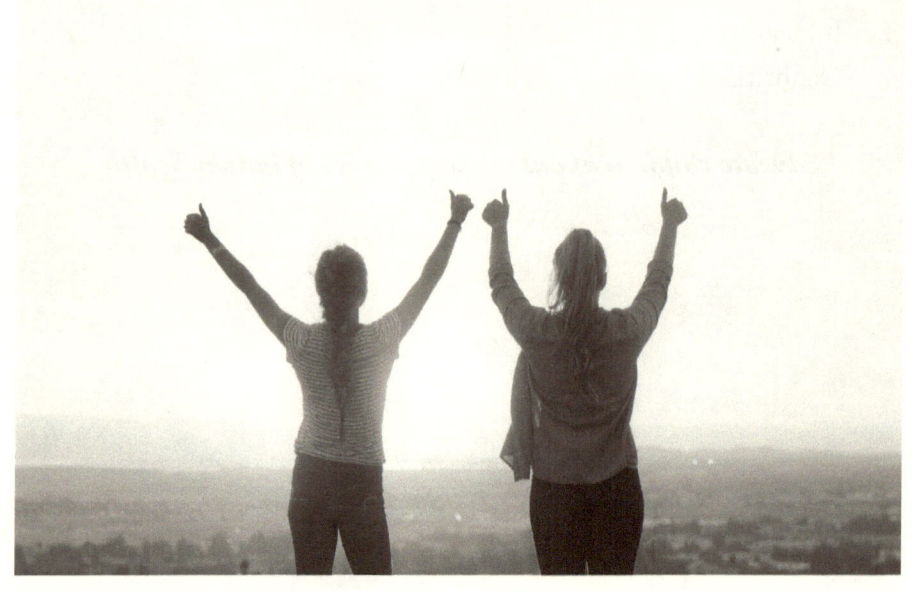

"A woman's health is her capital."

– Harriet Beecher Stowe
(American abolitionist and author)

"When women take care of their health they become their best friend."

– Maya Angelou (Poet)

I would like to share the story of a female patient in her forties afflicted by kidney dysfunction we encountered recently. A doctor friend of mine called over to me and shifted this patient from his secondary care centre.

I received the patient an hour later with puffy face and swollen legs. She didn't have diabetes or hypertension or any major hospitalisation previously. The urinary bag was hanging by the side of the cot. The accompanying person revealed that there was low urine output for the past two days.

She was completely normal a week back and didn't recollect having fever or urinary symptoms. I went through her investigation reports.

I knew her kidneys were deteriorating rapidly. If not intervened at the earliest it may go to a point of no return. It could not be cured by an operation or a single dose of a magic drug. Medications needed to be started without waiting for the test results.

We started the medications and supportive therapy to decrease the swelling and increase the urine output. Luckily she started to respond. Her creatinine value which was on the rise in the initial two days of admission started to plateau.

Kidney biopsy, a test that involves taking tissue out from the kidney to aid in accurate diagnosis was done swiftly. The patient continued to improve and her kidney function trended towards normal over the next 10 days of her hospital stay.

Her kidney biopsy report arrived. It revealed that her kidney is being affected by a disease that commonly affects women than men – Systemic Lupus Erythematosus.

Many other diseases afflict women disproportionately, most of them have gloomy implications.

Nature

Nature postpones vascular disease like a heart attack for women mostly by virtue of the female hormones. But that is not true for kidney disease. Due to their hormonal and chromosomal nature, a few kidney diseases occur almost exclusively in women.

The systemic lupus erythematosus (SLE)

SLE is a disease that affects many organs including skin and kidneys. It is almost an exclusive disease of women. About 50% of people with SLE can develop kidney damage. If detected at an early stage, appropriate drugs will help to maintain the kidney function

Urinary tract infection

Women are more likely to be infected than men because of the varying anatomy of the urinary tract. This is due to the fact that the length of the urinary passage (urethra) is shorter in women.

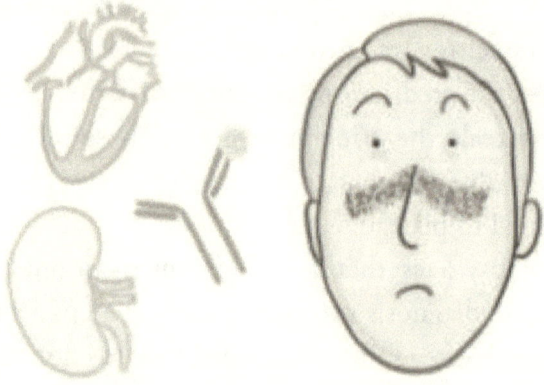

Urinary tract infection in pregnancy

Urinary tract infection occurring in pregnancy even without symptoms should be identified and treated to prevent detrimental effects on the mother and the growing foetus.

Hypertension in pregnancy

This disease is called Pre-Eclampsia. In advanced stages, it affects the kidneys. In this disease, protein is excreted in urine and there will be swelling of the feet. In some women, high blood pressure continues even after pregnancy and regular follow up is needed.

Kidney failure

Pregnancy also triggers a rare disease, hemolytic uremic syndrome. It may lead to permanent damage if not identified and treated early.

Cervical Cancer:

Cancer of the Cervix is one of the most common cancers in women. In advanced stages, it can cause obstruction to urine flow and result in renal failure.

Kidney care for women

Even in the modern era women don't have access to medical care compared to men in developing countries. It is also true for kidney diseases. This greatly hampers the detection and treatment of kidney diseases.

> *"Women should themselves take care of their kidney health as they take care of their children."*

As the Age Advances – Kidney Ailment in Elderly

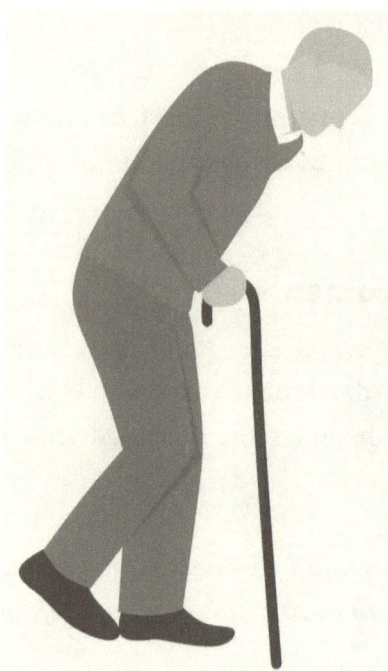

"Everybody's going to have some degree of health problems, as we get older. I think we've gotta maintain."

– Tom Hanks (Filmmaker)

I was ready to leave home at 6 pm from the hospital.

I got a call from the emergency department.

"Sir, one elderly male has come and has not passed urine since today morning. He also has severe lower abdomen pain."

I rushed to the ER.

A gentleman nearing his seventies was lying on the bed and wincing with pain. I gently examined his abdomen. The urinary bladder was full. There must be some blockage in the urinary tract.

We put a catheter and it drained around one and a half litre of urine. He was relieved of pain immediately. He was accompanied by his son. I discussed with both of them about his past symptoms. He has been having urinary symptoms for the past three months.

At his age, these are the typical symptoms of prostate gland enlargement which is a tiny gland encircling the outer urinary tube (urethra) in males. I ordered blood tests and imaging of the abdomen.

Prostate Gland

The prostate gland normally enlarges to some degree in all men as age advances. Few hormonal factors are also involved. The proportion of symptomatic individuals increases as age advances. It is considered a natural response of the body to ageing. More than half of men above 60 years may have this problem. Yearly examination is a must for elderly males to identify problems at an early stage

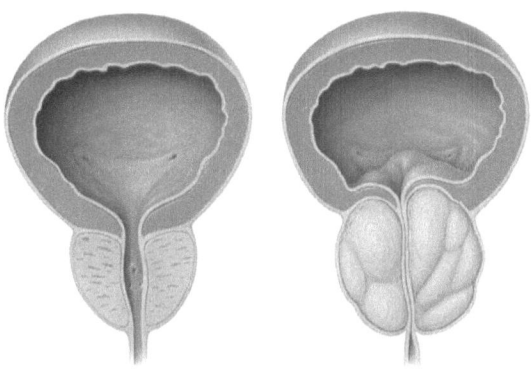

Normal Prostate   Enlarged Prostate

Symptoms
- Thin urinary stream
- Frequent urination especially at night time
- Dribbling of urine
- Sense of incomplete urination
- Most elderly people accommodate to the symptoms and don't seek medical care

Remedies
Lifestyle changes
- Avoiding more fluids just before bedtime
- Avoiding beverages that increase urinary frequency (coffee, alcohol)
- After urinating, wait for few minutes and then void again (Double voiding)

How to avoid progressive enlargement of the prostate?
- Knowledge of symptoms and medical consult at the earliest
- Drugs when required

Need for surgery
- When medicine doesn't control symptoms
- Enlargement is progressive
- Urinary stasis
- Kidney dysfunction

Prostate enlargement doesn't mean prostate cancer, though we screen these patients for cancer at regular intervals.

Prostate Cancer
It is much less common than the prostate gland enlargement described above. Here early detection and appropriate therapy will portend complete cure.

Other kidney problems in elderly people

As age advances renal function declines which is physiological and does not necessarily need specific treatment. Chronic diseases like diabetes and hypertension are common in the elderly and due to these risk factors, they may have kidney problems.

Urinary incontinence

Urinary incontinence is involuntary passage or urgency to urinate. It is common in the elderly due to weakened nerves supplying the urinary bladder. It can cause problems like urinary tract infections.

Most regard this as a part of normal ageing and ignore the symptoms completely. Measures can be taken to minimize this problem.

- Reducing liquids two to three hours before bedtime
- Cutting down food or drinks that make the symptoms worse
- Reducing alcohol, caffeine, spicy and acidic foods
- Keeping the blood sugar under control if you have diabetes

In persistent urinary incontinence – Remedies

Medications – That relaxes the urinary bladder

Surgery – In extreme cases, to repair the tissues that support the urinary bladder

Are you caring for the elderly?

- Elders should be repeatedly reminded of the symptoms of their kidney diseases.
- After 40 years of age, a **PSA** test should be done yearly to identify prostate cancer in the early stage.
- Be aware of their drug intake as the adverse effect on the kidneys will be more pronounced in the elderly.

> *"Always remember that elders are more prone to kidney insult. Early intervention is better."*

Remember, Drugs Can Do Harm to the Kidneys

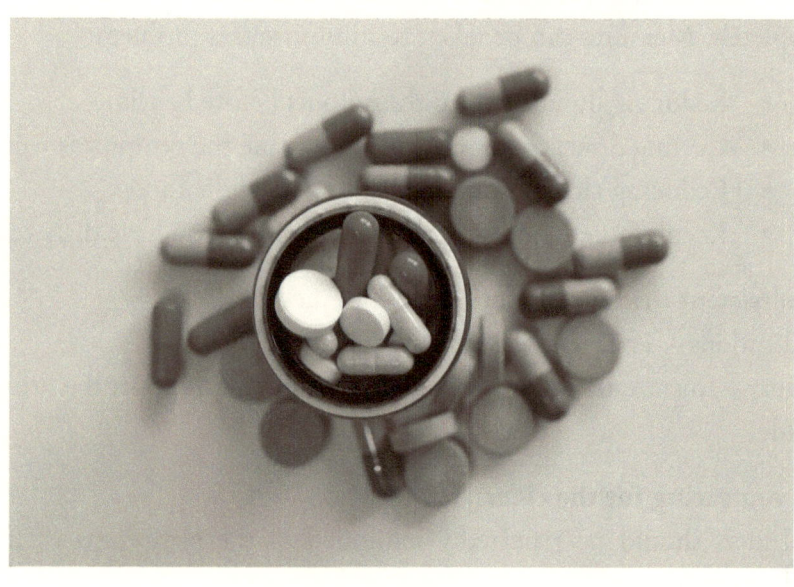

"For the chemistry that works on one patient, May not work for the next Because even Medicine has its own conditions."

– Suzy Kassem (MAXIMS OF MEDICINE)

At the Airport, when I was in the waiting lounge, an elderly man came over to me,

"Doctor, How are you?"

I could remember him well.

He was my patient whom I saw a year earlier.

He took self-medication for arthritis and landed in acute kidney failure. He required two sessions of dialysis. He recovered well after a few days. He then consulted me a couple of times to follow up and was doing well. I then referred him to a specialist for his arthritis.

He had a person accompanying him. Pointing to him he said, "Doctor, this is my friend. He has the habit of taking painkillers for frequent arthritis pain. Please tell him about the effects of harmful drugs."

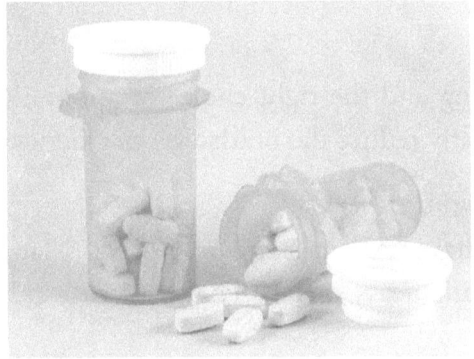

Why kidneys?
Even though the two kidneys together make up about 0.5% of the body weight, about 25% of the body's blood circulates to the kidneys. This is for the kidneys to clean up the metabolic waste products of the body.

By virtue of this, the kidney is the main organ affected by any harmful drugs, chemicals or poison.

Why are some drugs harmful?
Depending on the potency of the drug and its chemical structure the extent of the kidney damage is variable with each drug.

Who is more prone to the effects of the drugs?
- Older people
- Diabetic patients
- Patients who have pre-existing kidney dysfunction
- Patients with cardiac ailments
- Patients with dehydration

Most often the damage may be reversible but occasionally kidney damage ensues. However, most prescribed medications are safe in kidney disease as long as the doctor makes special changes to the dosage.

Caution in a few groups of drugs
Pain relievers
It doesn't cause harm to all individuals. But to a susceptible individual, even one dose can harm the kidneys.

Some antibiotics
Appropriate dosing and the right choice of antibiotic for a particular infection will greatly reduce the burden on the kidneys.

Some traditional medicines
Not all traditional medicines are approved. Many such contains impurities including heavy metals. They can cause kidney failure.

Few chemotherapy drugs
Your doctor will take the necessary precautions to prevent kidney injury due to cancer chemotherapy drugs. Periodic monitoring is warranted for certain drugs.

These are the common drugs, but other groups of drugs can also affect the kidneys.

What are the impacts on the kidneys?
- Acute kidney failure
- Chronic kidney failure
- Protein in urine
- High blood pressure

How can you prevent it?
Do not take any medication without doctor's advice.

People with diabetes, the elderly and those taking other medications should be more vigilant.

Kidney failure in hospitalised patients
Among patients admitted to the intensive care unit, about 25% of them have kidney ailment during admission. Of them, people with early kidney failure are completely reversible once the preceding illness improves.

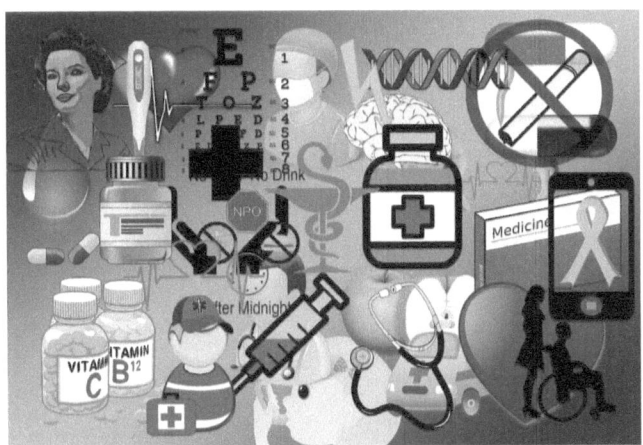

Causes:
- Multi-organ dysfunction
- Infection
- Shock – Persistent low blood pressure.
- Drugs
- Dehydration
- Contrast dyes

Avoidance methods: Watchful observation
The medical team caring for the patient will take utmost precautions to reduce kidney damage. But due to the interplay of multiple factors, renal failure can be inevitable.

PART 2

Kidney Failure and Treatment

Kidney Attack – Acute Kidney Failure

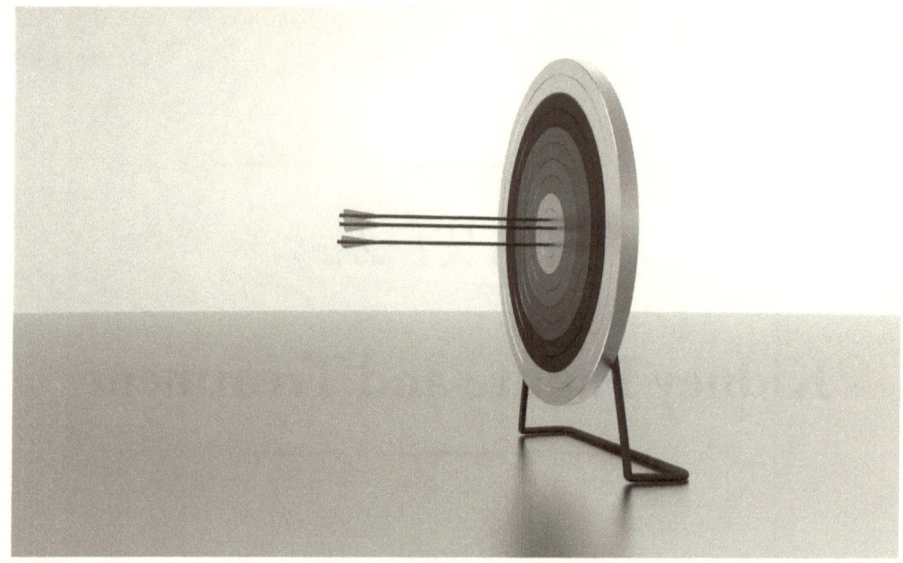

"Let the physician enquire into the nature of the disease, its cause and its method of cure and treat it faithfully according to medical rule."

– THIRUKKURAL 948

My friend Raghav rushed to my cabin on a Monday morning.

"My son Naveen had fever for a week. I admitted him to a hospital near my home. Three days back, his eyes looked yellow and urine output was less. Since yesterday, there is swelling of his feet. I am totally afraid. Shall I bring him here?"

In an hour Naveen was brought to our hospital in a stretcher. He was struggling to breathe. His legs were swollen and his eyes appeared bright yellow.

I had a glance over his test results. His blood creatinine level was 5.6 mg/dl. From my analysis, I concurred that he will require dialysis. I ordered the nurses to prepare him for dialysis and took Raghav aside for a conversation regarding the disease state.

"Does he need dialysis at present?" Raghav asked.

"Currently, he definitely requires dialysis. For him the kidney failure is temporary. Don't worry, It is curable." I consoled him.

I tried to explain about acute renal failure to my friend.

Just like a heart attack, this type of kidney failure can be called a kidney attack.

It is important to identify and treat them early to prevent acute complications and chronic failure.

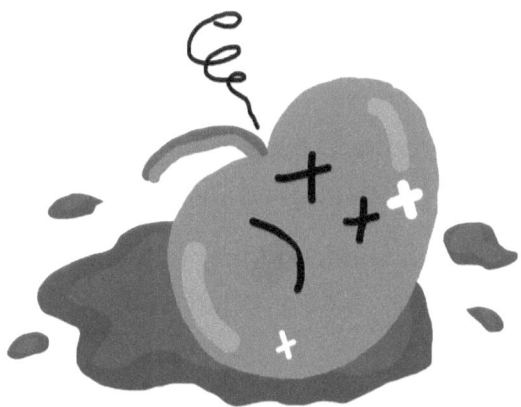

Causes

What causes acute kidney failure?
1. Decreased blood flow to the kidneys (blood loss, burns, heart failure)
2. Fever (malaria, leptospirosis, etc.)
3. Profuse diarrhoea and vomiting
4. Urinary tract infections
5. Bloodborne infections (sepsis)
6. Some medications (pain relievers, antibiotics, etc.)
7. Toxic Bites (Snakebite)
8. Some diseases in pregnancy
9. Urinary tract obstruction (Prostate gland enlargement/Stones)
10. Diseases directly affecting the kidneys

Other symptoms

What are the symptoms of this kidney attack? Can you explain it?
- The urine quantity may be low
- Shortness of breath (Flooding of lungs with fluid)
- At times 50% of kidney fails before being detected by blood tests
- Diminished food intake
- Mental confusion

Basic cause

The problem which has caused kidney failure is more important. It is essential to find out the basic cause and address it.

What is the treatment for sudden kidney failure?
Not all patients with acute kidney failure will require dialysis. The need for dialysis depends on the nature and severity of kidney dysfunction. A Nephrologist will identify and treat the disease that has caused kidney failure. Fluid and diet have to be taken as per the doctor's advice.

Does dialysis need to be continued indefinitely?
Dialysis treatment may be discontinued once the kidney damage begins to recover.

Rarely, if kidney dysfunction persists over three to four weeks then kidney tissue (kidney biopsy) testing may be required.

Vulnerable people for acute kidney failure
- Aged persons
- Diabetes mellitus
- Hypertension
- Cardiac patients

Sent home..
Fifteen days later, Naveen was free from dialysis. All the tubes were removed.

He was fit for discharge.

"Is he fully fit for discharge? Any other follow up tests required?"

"Yes, his kidney function is restored to the normal state. But you may have to carry out these simple tests once in three to six months."

- Blood pressure
- Urine test
- Creatinine in the blood

He was happy and thankful while leaving the hospital.

"Timely intervention saves kidney and life in acute kidney failure."

Chronic Kidney Failure

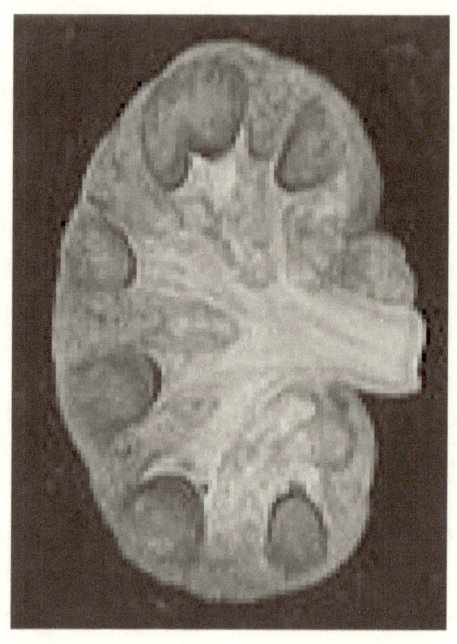

It was 9'o clock in the morning, I sat down afresh and asked my secretary to send the first patient of the day.

A man in his early fifties, lean with sparse hair on the scalp came up to me. He looked anxious. He was sent by my friend who is a general physician in the nearby town.

I made him a bit relaxed and enquired regarding his family and job pattern, as for any other patients. He was a manager in a textile firm.

He started "Doctor I had a master health check-up in my company. They told me my creatinine level in the blood was 2.1 mg. His face showed an expression as if the whole world is doomed. Then I went to two more doctors and checked in other labs too. The report was 1.8 mg and 2 mg in other labs. I don't know what to do now."

He was almost crying.

I held his palms and the soothing effect was revealed on his face. He got relaxed a little.

I tried to convince him that there may be minor differences in creatinine levels, depending on the timing of the tests and diet. Laboratory variations also count.

I saw his entire report thoroughly including an ultrasound of the kidneys. I was convinced he had Chronic Kidney Disease, meaning kidney damage that cannot be reversed to a larger extent.

I tried to figure out what factors would have damaged the kidneys. He never had diabetes or high blood pressure.

"It is true that your kidneys are affected. But it is impossible to ascertain at this point, what would have caused it!" I said in a normal tone.

He screamed at me in an explosive voice.

"Doctor, for heaven's sake cure me. I will take whatever medicine you prescribe. I can also undergo a kidney transplant to get back my kidney function fully. My spouse has the same blood group as mine."

It took a bit of my time to console him.

"Keep yourself relaxed first. Although your kidney failure is chronic it is still in the early stage. First, you have to realize that your kidney function or creatinine levels cannot be restored completely. Progression varies from few months to more than 20 years depending on the quality of the kidneys. It should also be borne in mind that not all people with permanent kidney disease need dialysis or kidney transplantation."

I tried to explain him in detail regarding chronic kidney disease.

People who are more prone to chronic kidney failure
Common Causes
- Diabetes mellitus
- Hypertension
- Hereditary diseases (Polycystic kidney disease)
- Glomerulonephritis/Nephrotic Syndrome
- Kidney stone disease
- Obstructive kidney disease
- Some rare diseases

How severe is my kidney failure?
Kidney failure is graded by the filtration capacity known as GFR.

It is a calculated value ascertained from the creatinine value in the blood. It roughly denotes your kidney function in percentage.

Stage of failure	Level	GFR (ml/min/1.73 m^2)
The first stage	I	> 90 with other abnormalities
The second stage	II	60 – 89
The third stage	III	30 – 59
Fourth level	IV	15 – 29
Fifth level	V	< 15

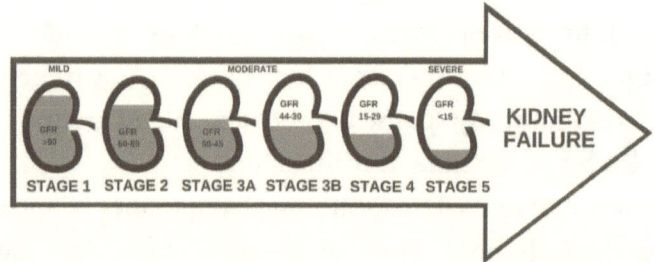

"Doctor, if I have kidney damage then my urine quantity should have been reduced. I also don't have any swelling of my feet."

The initial stages usually don't produce any symptoms. It is usually incidentally detected during routine health check-ups, urine examinations or blood tests done during other illnesses.

What are other signs of early-stage renal failure?
- Physical fatigue
- Anemia
- Hypertension
- Swelling of feet and face
- Decreased urine volume
- Frequent urination during the night

"What can I do now, Doctor?"
GFR calculation reveals that your kidney damage is in the third stage (STAGE-3.)

Our treatment can delay or prevent you from moving to the dialysis stage for many years.

"You need not worry."

I sent him back with drugs and lifestyle advice with a hope that my words would have made him think positively.

"Early-stage kidney dysfunction can occur without symptoms. Follow up with the doctor as advised. Patient participation is vital in preventing the progression of the disease."

When End-Stage Kidney Disease Strikes

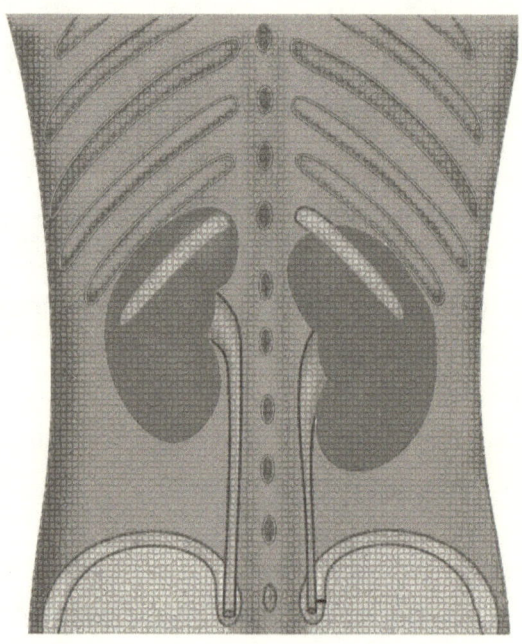

"When the kidneys fail to manufacture the proper kind of blood neither bone, muscle, gland nor brain can carry on."

– Homer William Smith

The emergency ward was unusually calm that day and I was spending my free time engaging with the general internists of our hospital.

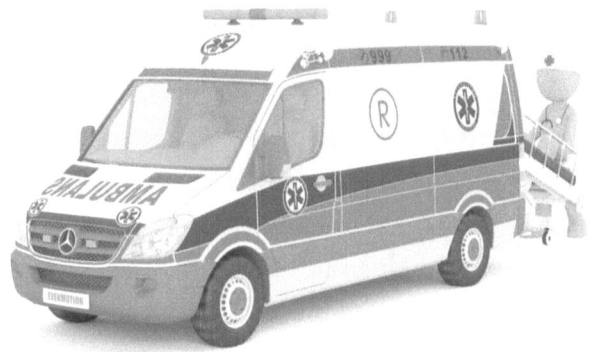

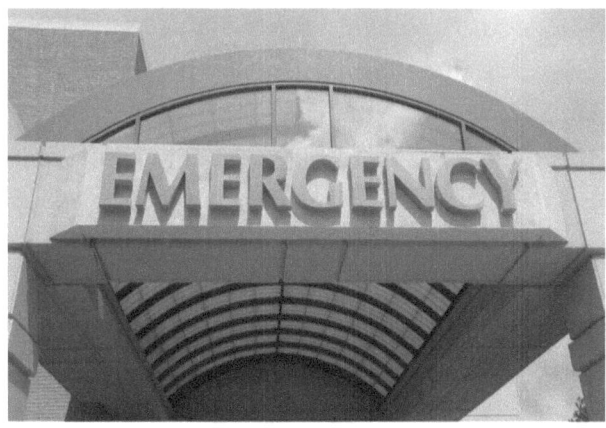

I heard the sound of the ambulance outside. A man nearing his sixties and grossly obese was brought inside, face unshaven and puffy. He was only slightly responsive.

He was breathing at a rate of 40 breaths per minute as to the normal rate of 15 per minute. I rushed him to the resuscitation bay, kept a tight mask approximating the mouth and nose. The monitor was connected as his heart rate showed 40 per minute and blood pressure galloping at 190/100 mm Hg. Both his legs were swollen up to the thigh and his lungs were flooded with fluid. The senior nurse started to load calcium as soon as she saw the cardiac monitor, even before the blood investigations revealed increased potassium, which could stop the heart at any time. She used her logical thinking at that point.

Another nurse was quick to put the venflon, drew the blood for investigation and gave diuretics, a drug that expels the urine out and reduces lung congestion.

The blood gas values returned by the time and showed a potassium value of 8.8, which is almost double the normal value. His heart may stop any time now. Blood values around 6 are common in untreated kidney failure patients but this value is rarely compatible with life and they succumb to cardiac arrest while at home or during transit.

There are a few measures to decrease the potassium levels temporarily and stabilise the heart. But ultimately excess potassium must be filtered out from the blood artificially by a process called dialysis.

Few boluses of calcium were pushed into him along with consecutive doses of salbutamol nebulisation. As a physician, you are forced to act briskly in such situations as it is a life-threatening emergency.

I ordered the house officers to shift him to the intensive care unit for further stabilisation and wanted to know about the patient's past health status from his family.

I summoned the relatives of the patient who were apprehensive but fully aware of what was going on inside, seeing the urgency of our paramedics. I briefly explained that he needed intensive care and immediate dialysis. His condition was stable compared to the state in which he was brought to the hospital.

He was rushed into the ICU, his respiratory muscles fatigued and the mask was ineffective to support his respiration. A tube was slid into his tracheal lumen and connected to a ventilator.

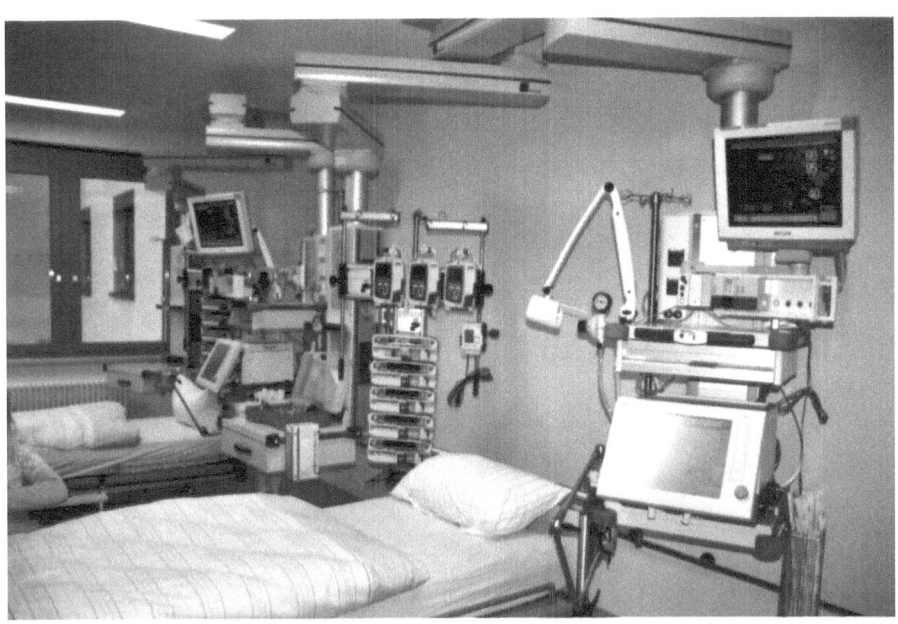

A dialysis catheter was inserted into a large vein going into the heart and its tip was confirmed to be in the right side chamber of the heart. He was initiated on dialysis, a process that clears his metabolic waste products and potassium from the bloodstream. His kidneys have become ineffective in removing them.

All our efforts were done in less than thirty minutes and a well-co-ordinated team is essential to carry out these processes smoothly and without any error.

I was happy that he was out of danger and handed over the patient to the intensive care team. By the time I got the initial reports, it revealed his urea level was 235 mg/dl and creatinine was 14 mg/dl, alarmingly high levels.

He was diagnosed to have chronic kidney disease around five years back at an early stage. He was also prescribed medications. He assumed that a lot of medications will damage the kidneys further and stopped everything. He took only blood pressure medications on and off and never attempted to visit a kidney specialist.

I explained this to the family members. "This is end-stage kidney disease for sure. The harmful substances and toxins are affecting every organ and cell of his body. This state – could have been prevented if he had consulted and taken the advice of his doctor regularly."

We had daily rounds and discussed the course of the patient with his family members. We were happy with his progress after admission.

The patient came out of the intensive care unit after five days, fully tired but willing to cooperate for further treatment.

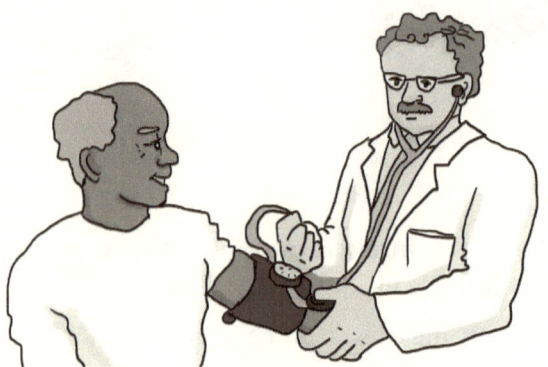

Symptoms of End-Stage kidney disease
- Excessive fluid accumulation in lungs, shortness of breath
- Decreased Urine output
- Fluid accumulation over the feet and around the eyes.
- Tiredness
- Decreased food intake/vomiting
- Bone pain or bone fracture
- Altered consciousness
- Sleep disturbances
- Chest pain
- Itching

Since the toxins affect all parts of the body, it can cause symptoms related to any organ. Few patients may be devoid of any symptoms.

Differences in regular and irregular treatment for chronic kidney disease
Example

X	Y
Who does not take appropriate treatment for kidney failure	One who is on regular follow up for kidney failure
Kidney disease progresses faster	Illness controlled over the long term
Dialysis being started on an emergency basis	Can avoid dialysis or delay the onset of end-stage disease
Cost and burden of intensive care unit	No
May need to face complications such as infections & heart ailments	No

When to start dialysis in end-stage kidney disease?
Do all these patients need dialysis?

Your doctor is the best person to decide the time of initiation of dialysis based on symptoms and laboratory values. Not all persons progressing to the end-stage will need dialysis urgently. It will be decided based upon one's symptoms and extent of kidney dysfunction as evident in blood values.

> *"If end-stage kidney disease strikes, strengthen courage, make a plan and execute effectively."*

How to Postpone Dialysis?

"Individuals with kidney disease who are able to obtain treatment early experience a higher quality of life and are able to maintain more of their day-to-day activities, including keeping their jobs."

– Xavier Becerra (American politican)

There are a few simple steps that will help one avoid or postpone dialysis after being diagnosed with chronic kidney disease. They are both important for the caretaker as well as the patient.

It should be remembered that kidney failure management is not a one-time affair as like an antibiotic course for a bacterial infection or appendicectomy for the inflamed appendix. It is a continuous process.

Understand the Disease and Plan

Get a very thorough knowledge of the disease in whatever way you can. Assess what stage of chronic kidney disease you are in. Discuss with your Nephrologist about the way forward and the frequency of check-ups. Get clarified regarding the disease during the initial stage of the disease itself. Research has shown that in patients who are well engaged in management, the progression of the disease is slower.

Anemia

Anemia indicates a low hemoglobin level in your blood and denotes the extent of decreased oxygenation to the tissues. Correction and restoration of hemoglobin to the optimal level are important as anemia worsens the existing kidney dysfunction.

Watch your minerals

Control of mineral balance is important in early-stage kidney failure itself. Deranged phosphorus and uric acid levels will worsen kidney failure. Your Nephrologist will also prescribe Alkali to decrease the acid load to the kidneys. These parameters need to be monitored periodically.

Protein intake

Protein intake in early kidney failure should be modest. Very low intake may lead to nutritional deficiency whereas overtly high intake will cause an increased burden on the kidneys and will accelerate kidney failure.

Lifestyle measures

The importance of lifestyle measures like exercise, pranayama and yoga are additive to your other efforts. They should always form parts of the treatment plan.

High blood pressure

High blood pressure may be a cause or the result of kidney failure. Whatever may be, uncontrolled high blood pressure accelerates kidney dysfunction. You should be on appropriate drugs that decrease the blood pressure effectively and do good to the kidneys.

Blood sugar level

It is a well known fact that blood sugar control gains paramount importance if you are a diabetic and have kidney failure. A comprehensive care plan for diabetic control replenishes the kidneys.

Watch for change in symptoms

Any change or unusual symptoms denote worsening kidney failure and early intervention is needed.

No unnecessary drugs

Caution should be maintained when taking over the counter drugs or when taking drugs for other ailments.

Positive thoughts

Always be in a positive frame of mind regarding the illness. We cannot change the past but definitely can adopt healthy practices for further well being.

Diet

Analyse the diet which will suit you the best. The pros and cons of various diet plans need to be discussed. Nephrologist and a renal dietician, both are core members of your diet planning.

Weight reduction

If a chronic kidney disease patient is obese, weight reduction will be of great favour for the kidneys.

Know your medications

Your doctor will prescribe various medications to tackle different components of kidney disease. Try to know about each of them. Discuss the newer drugs which would potentially slow the kidney disease.

The readers are advised to refer to other chapters to know in detail about the preventive measures.

People with early stage renal failure

	Do'S	Don't S
1	Getting to know yourself and your caregivers fully about your kidneys and their functions	Failure to go to the doctor when dehydrated
2	Complete control of the probable cause of renal failure	Consumption of unauthorized drugs
3	Diet • Exercise • Drug • Periodic tests	Neglecting mild symptoms
4	Blood pressure control	
5	Self-help	
6	Vaccination	

Model diet plan for patients with chronic kidney disease – (Not on dialysis)

6 am:	Skimmed Milk – 100 ml (without sugar)
8 am:	Idly – 2/Dosa – 2/Idiappam – 2/Wheat uppuma – ½ cup Sambar – 1 cup
10 am:	Vegetable Salad – 1 cup (Cucumber) Fruit – 100g (Apple/Guava/Papaya)
12.30 pm:	Rice – ¾ cup (Raw weight – 75g)/Chapatthi – 2 Vegetable Gravy – 1 cup Vegetable Porial – ½ cup, Buttermilk – 1 cup (50ml)
4 pm:	Skimmed Milk – 100 ml (without sugar) Whole Pulses – ¼ cup (50gm)
7.30 pm:	Idly – 2/Dosa – 2/Idiappam – 2/Wheat Uppuma – ½ cup Vegetable Gravy – 1 cup or onion chutney 150ml
9.30 pm:	Skimmed Milk – 100ml (without sugar) Total Calories: 1600kcal/day Total protein: 40gm/day

"A comprehensive plan and approach are needed to avoid or postpone dialysis. Look into all aspects of management which would fetch you reaping benefits. Lots of nutritional information, books, alternative medicine are available in the market to avoid dialysis. Caution should be exercised in following them. Trust your doctor and take his advice."

Cleansing the Blood – Dialysis

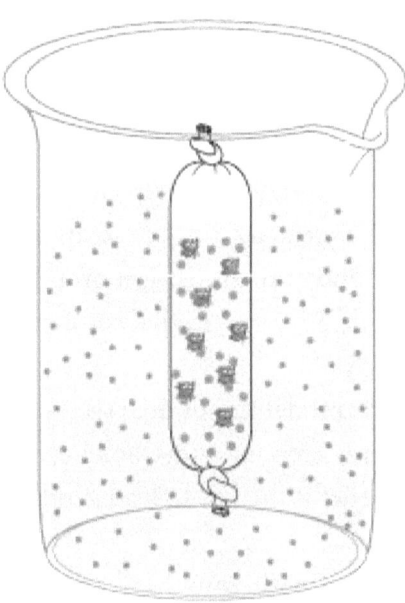

"The dialysis lets the patient live a close to normal life so they can be a grandparent or go to work."

– Nora Daludado

> *"If a problem is fixable, if a situation is such that you can do something about it, then there is no need to worry."*
>
> **– Dalai Lama**

As we have already seen, end-stage kidney disease is not an end-stage by itself. Yes, the kidneys have reached the point of no return. The function of the kidneys has to be substituted by some modalities.

As a Nephrologist, I have discussed in leaps and bounds with the patients and caregivers with regard to the management of terminal stage dysfunction of this vital organ in the human body.

An infinite number of questions may arise in one's mind after getting this diagnosis.

"Should I depend on the machine for the rest of my life? What are the implications on my profession, family, financial and spiritual life?"

Adapting one's lifestyle accordingly and approaching the diagnosis in the right frame of mind is the most important aspect of the dialysis procedure itself. Successful long term dialysis is possible from newborn babies to the very elderly.

Understanding the modalities of dialysis, taking the pros and cons of each one of them into account and wholeheartedly choosing one of them without any disbelief is the key to lead a long life and allay the fear of dialysis.

Clarifying the doubts with your Nephrologist along the course of decision making is of utmost importance. The modern era offers many more choices of renal replacement therapy which has vastly improved the quality of life and one can convert the disadvantage to an optimistic engagement.

Purpose of dialysis

Dialysis – Greek "To separate or dissolve"

Toxins and waste products start to accumulate at least months to years before the kidneys have fully failed. Dialysis is a treatment that does most, if not all of the things normally done by healthy kidneys. Dialysis is needed when your kidneys do not work well enough to keep you healthy.

Dialysis removes waste products, salt and extra water to prevent them from building up in the body; it helps in maintaining a safe level of certain chemicals in blood such as potassium, sodium, bicarbonate, calcium and phosphorous and also aids to control blood pressure.

Blood purification machine (Hemodialysis)

Hemodialysis is the method of renal replacement therapy followed by more than 80% of patients requiring dialysis.

Blood is extracted, passed into a dialysis filter and sent back to the body. The dialyser contains thousands of micro filters, the outer surface of which is bathed by commercial dialysis fluid. While the blood passes through these micro filters the toxins are removed by the conventional process of osmosis.

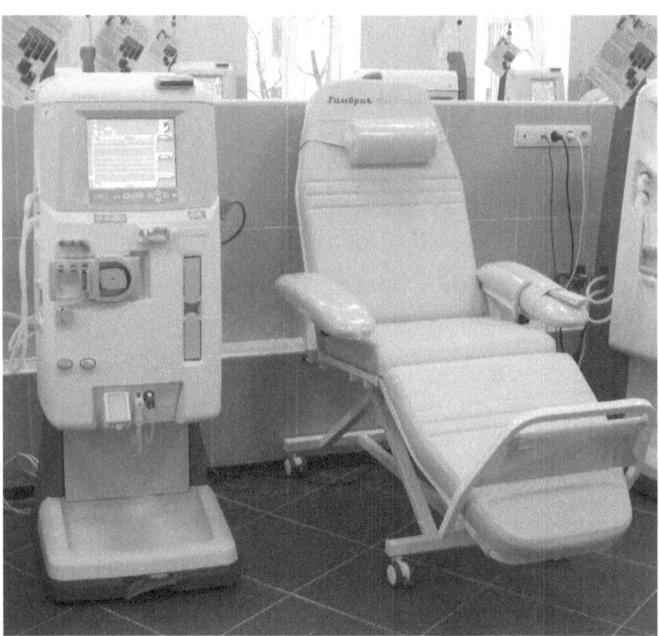

Dialysis machine

Dialysis is a complex treatment that takes time to understand. Symptoms may be different for each patient at the start of dialysis.

How and when is the dialysis initiated?

For those who are in urgent need of this treatment, a flexible tube is inserted in the neck. Blood will be drawn through the catheter by the blood pump in the dialysis machine. The dialysed blood is then returned to the body through the same tube.

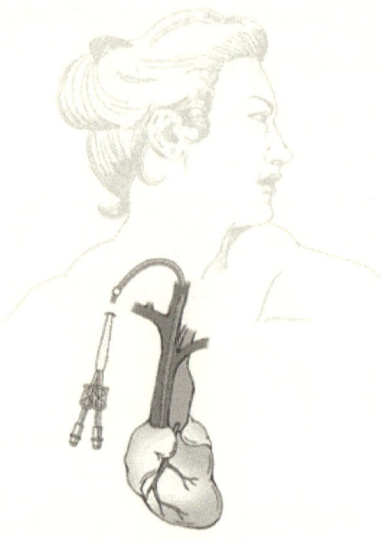

The role of Arteriovenous fistula

The best way to perform hemodialysis is to have a fistula from which blood can be drawn to the dialysis machine and sent back to the body. There are fewer and negligible infective complications with AV fistula.

AV FISTULA – What is it?

Two blood vessels are joined by a minor surgical procedure. It takes six to eight weeks to mature and be usable. The blood is drawn with the help of a needle, passes through the dialyser and returned via another needle. There are some simple safety measures that should be followed as advised by your doctor.

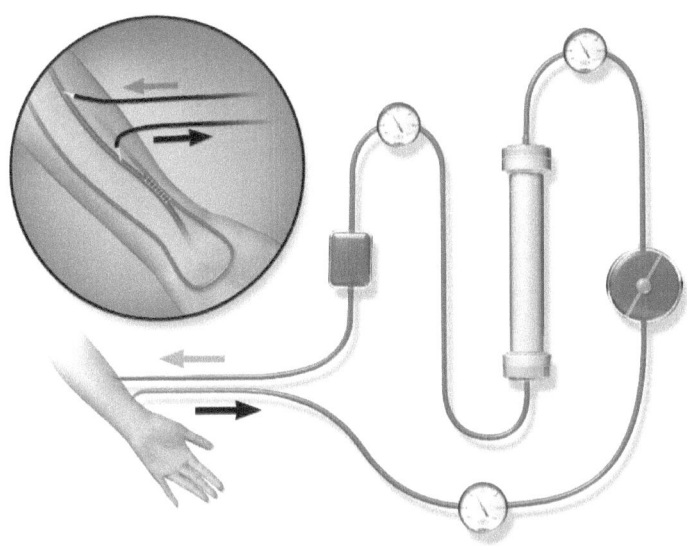

Fistula – Utmost importantce
Patients are taught to observe the thrill of the fistula. If they notice any undue bleeding or decrease in the thrill they should contact the dialysis centre immediately.

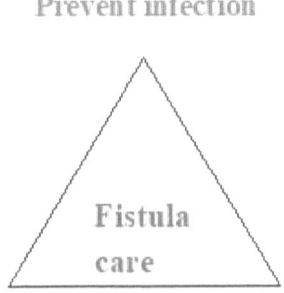

AV Graft–
In individuals without suitable blood vessels for AV fistula, synthetic grafts can be implanted from which blood can be drawn.

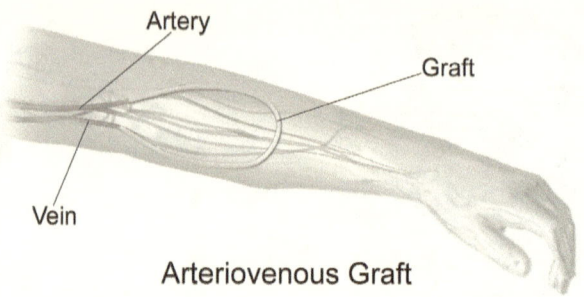

Arteriovenous Graft

Tunnelled Catheter

It is an option for patients in whom AVfistula and AV graft are not feasible. This type of catheter can be used for a longer period of time.

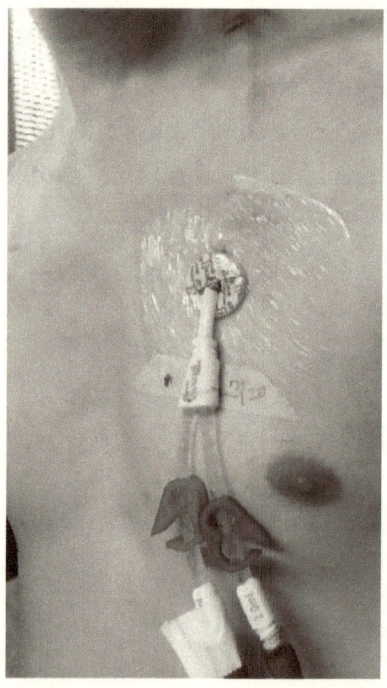

How many times hemodialysis should be done?
Two or three times a week. One needs to spend four hours in the hospital. Generally, more number of sessions per week is good to get rid of the toxins.

How much fluids will be removed during each session of dialysis?
By physical examination and some simple tests, your Nephrologist will decide on how much fluid should be removed during each dialysis session.

Few disadvantages of hemodialysis
- Frequent visits to a dialysis centre.
- During the treatment, some people may develop a drop in blood pressure.
- Some may develop fatigue after treatment.
- Muscle cramps/headaches may occur.

These can be easily managed with lifestyle modification and discussion with the caregivers. Interactions with other patients and caregivers reduces stress.

Warning signs during hemodialysis
- Pain or bleeding in the fistula
- Chest pain
- Palpitation

Can this treatment be done at home?
Home hemodialysis is available and widespread in developed countries. Patients can do it themselves after adequate training.

Peritoneal Dialysis – CAPD

This is another type of dialysis therapy. Our abdomen has a membrane lined between the skin and the internal organs. It is called the peritoneal cavity. Letting fluid in and out of the peritoneal cavity requires a pipe-like system.

Methods

A minor procedure is done to put a soft, flexible plastic tube called a catheter into the belly. Most peritoneal dialysis catheters are placed in the lower abdomen. The dialysis treatment can be started two weeks after catheter placement.

The dialysate bag containing fluid has various mineral compositions. Dialysis fluid is instilled into the abdomen through the catheter. Waste products from the blood are absorbed by the dialysis fluid. When the fluid is drained out, it takes the waste and extra fluid out of the body. It takes about 20-30 minutes to drain the fluid in and out. Changing the bags is done manually about three to four times per day.

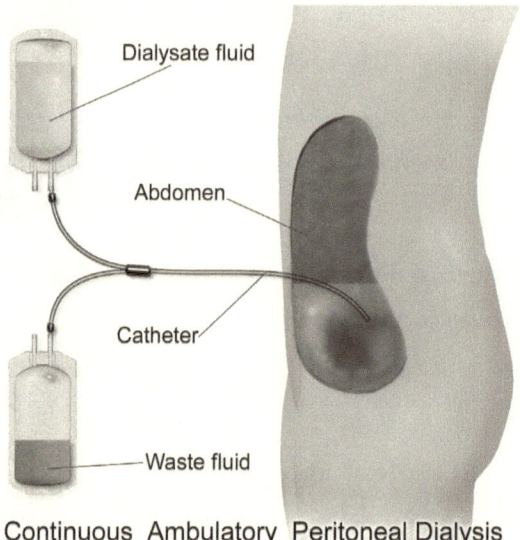

Continuous Ambulatory Peritoneal Dialysis

Advantages

- No frequent hospital visits
- Can be done even in remote places
- Avoids cross infection
- Suitable for executives and students
- Fluid intake can be liberal
- Sense of well being is better than hemodialysis
- Heart disease patients do better with peritoneal dialysis
- It is a very good mode of therapy when some kidney function is still present

Precautions

- Adequate replacement for protein losses should be done.
- Insulin dose may increase slightly in diabetics.
- Weight gain if any should be addressed.
- Risk of infection, if steps in changing bags are not followed correctly.
- Constipation should be prevented.
- Report to the doctor if you have fever, abdomen pain or altered colour of dialysate fluid.

APD Treatment (Automated Peritoneal Dialysis)

When the fluid exchange is done by machine overnight it is called APD (Automated Peritoneal Dialysis) which takes place for eight hours overnight and needs 30 minutes to set up and clean the machine before and after each session.

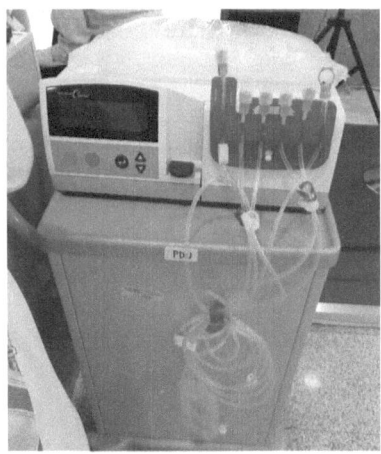

What are the treatment options?

How to choose a dialysis centre?
- Is it supervised by a dialysis trained physician or Nephrologist?
- Are there facilities for 24-hour emergency assistance?
- What are the opinions of other patients on dialysis at that centre?

- How are infection control practices handled?
- Are there isolation practices?

How to avoid infections in dialysis patients?
Vaccination

Appropriate vaccination to be done in the pre-dialysis period or after dialysis initiation.

- Hepatitis B (Viral disease affecting the liver)
- Varicella (To prevent chickenpox)
- Pneumococcal vaccine (To prevent pneumonia)
- Influenza vaccine (To prevent swine flu – yearly)

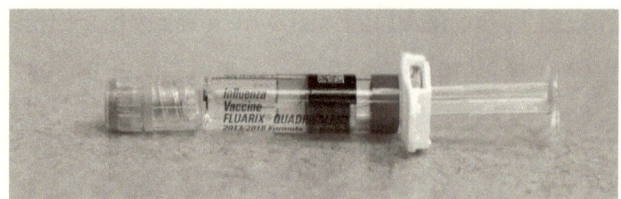

Dialysers

From a practical point of view using a single-use dialyser rather than reusable dialyser prevents cross-contamination and the spread of infection largely.

Dialysis mantra...

- Always try to maintain your ideal weight.
- Know your heart health.
- Supportive drugs are must.
- Regular tests in dialysis are important.
- Adequate nutrition and diet along with supplementation if required.

> *"Most other organ failures do not offer many choices for treatment. Kidney replacement therapy is unique in that it offers various choices to choose from."*

Getting a New Kidney – Kidney Transplantation

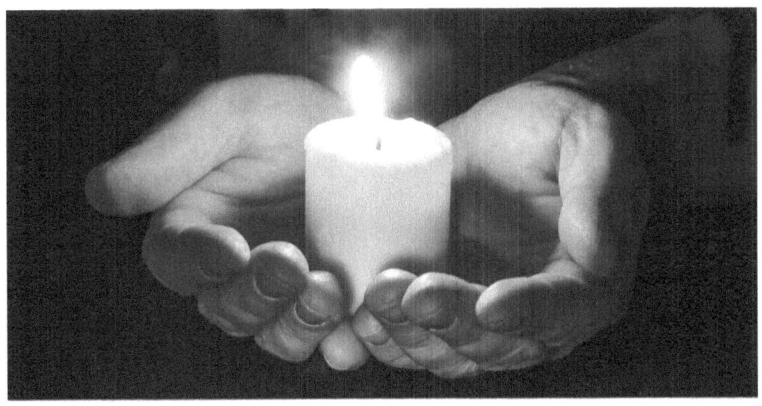

"Post-operatively the transplanted kidney functioned immediately with a dramatic improvement in the patient's renal and cardiopulmonary status. This spectacular success was a clear demonstration that organ transplantation could be life-saving."

– Joseph Murray (American plastic surgeon who performed the first successful human kidney transplant)

On a hot summer three years back, I happened to treat a young patient around 25 years of age.

On enquiry, he was symptomatic for the past two months with decreased weight and not taking the amount of food he used to be. His pants were loose and the shirts looked bigger for him. He was working in a software firm. In his college days, he was passionate about sports and was committed to academics. He didn't have any major illness in the past.

He had his basic tests done elsewhere and was referred to me. It was evident that he had end-stage kidney disease. I ordered a few other tests to confirm it and buy time to break the bad news to his parents. I received the investigation reports and began to discuss them with his parents.

You need to explain and give a vivid picture of the disease and its complications about what they think is a bleak situation. As Nephrologists, our day in and out passes with these patients with a failing organ. But for the caregivers, it is one and all for them and come to us with a ray of hope.

The parents already wore a worried look. I put to them straight, "This guy's kidneys are working with about less than 10% of its capacity."

"Doctor, how did it happen at a young age?" They asked with their heart pounding in anxiety.

They initially denied the facts before accepting and coming to terms.

"For a few patients, kidney disease progresses without any symptoms or there would have been minor symptoms that were ignored. He didn't have any symptoms that would have made early detection of kidney failure possible."

I tried to explain and convinced them that it is not a fault of them. Being in the end-stage, the exact cause of failure could not be ascertained.

"He requires some form of renal replacement therapy now. Renal transplantation alone will replace the kidney function naturally. He has to be prepared with a few dialysis sessions and to proceed with renal transplantation."

"Yes doctor, we can proceed with transplantation." Their voices now were a little loud and cheerful.

"Doctor, can you explain the whole process of renal transplantation?"

Who can donate?
- A person over 18 years of age
- Blood relative as a donor will be most appropriate
- The donor will be thoroughly examined by the physician
- Appropriate government authority should approve

Which blood type of kidney is acceptable?

Recipient (patient) Blood group	Donor Blood group
O	O
A	A, O
B	B, O
AB	A, B, O, AB

A positive or negative group is not a hindrance to transplantation. Kidney transplantation can also be performed with unmatched blood groups but needs extra preparation in the initial part and monitoring in the post-transplant period.

Donor

- The donor can lead a normal life after transplantation, one normally functioning kidney is good enough to eliminate waste products.
- Few tests will be carried on the donor.
- Diabetes/high blood pressure/cardiac/and Cancer patients will not be fit for kidney donation.
- The donor should be free of any infection.
- The ability to withstand surgery will be assessed.
- Related living donor poses a good genetic match.

Recipient

- Should have fairly normal heart function.
- Should be free from active infection.
- Should be fit for surgery.
- Appropriate vaccines should be given while waiting for the transplant.

Important

The transplant recipient and the donor should discuss with the doctor regarding the pros and cons. The shorter the time on dialysis, the better the longevity of the transplant.

Surgical method

1. Very rarely the patient's kidneys are removed.
2. The donor kidney's blood vessel will be joined to the recipient blood vessel and the donor ureter will be connected to the urinary bladder.
3. Total surgery duration may take four to six hours.
4. Will need to stay in the hospital for around seven to ten days.
5. The immediate function of a transplanted kidney denotes a successful outcome.

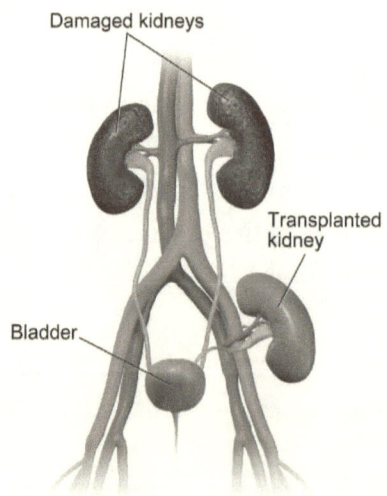

After kidney transplantation

- Medications are a must for maintaining the function of the transplanted kidney.
- Needs regular follow-up with the Nephrologist.
- The dose of medications will be reduced after the first year.
- Kidney biopsy may be required as per the treating Nephrologist's assessment.
- Monitoring is important.

"But doctor, we are a little scared," uttered the parents.

Don't be afraid! Thousands of kidney transplants are performed across the world.

The success rate of renal transplantation has increased over the last two decades.

Common medications

- Steroid – Prednisolone
- Cyclosporine/Tacrolimus
- Mycophenolate/Azathioprine

Along with this, some supportive medications should to be taken. The levels of the drug in the blood will be checked periodically.

Benefits of kidney transplantation

- Quality of life becomes better
- Water and dietary restriction can be relaxed
- Free from dialysis

Some precautions to follow after kidney transplantation

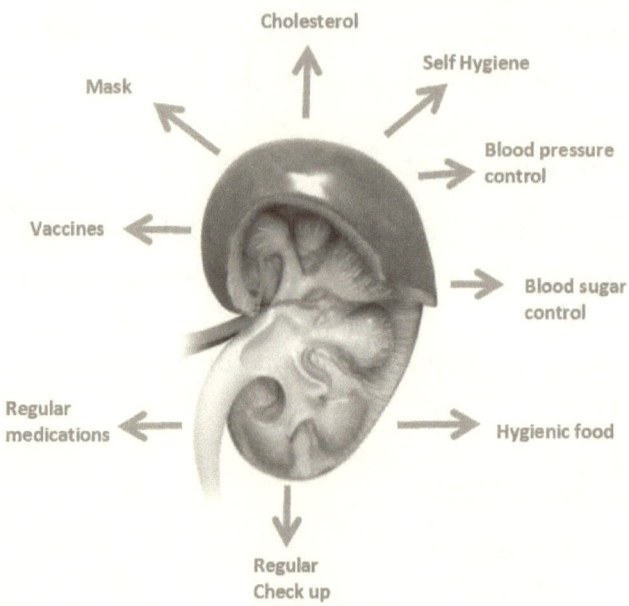

LIVING WELL AFTER KIDNEY TRANSPLANT

Physical activity

One should continue physical activity two to three months after renal transplant. This will prevent weight gain post-transplant.

Renal transplant is the only way to replace all the kidney functions and the best modality of treatment of end-stage kidney disease.

"We are born with two kidneys and only need one to survive. May be God gave us the other one so that we could give it away."

– Natalie Cole (Singer-Songwriter)

Kidney Beats – Getting Organ from a Brain Dead Donor

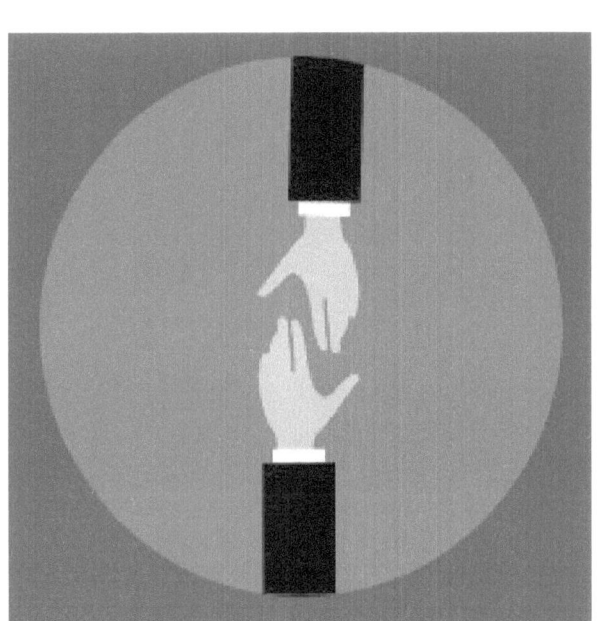

News of a young brain dead donor giving life to six organ failure patients was flashing on the television news on that holiday evening.

My thoughts went a few years back when I was a fellow in the Institute of Nephrology at the Madras Medical College, one of the largest centres treating kidney diseases.

That was the day, the national award-winning Tamil film editor Kishore suffered a stroke and was admitted to a private hospital in Chennai. It was unexpected given his age and health. The family was in utmost grief by the time he was brain dead. Any measure to treat was not going to bring him back

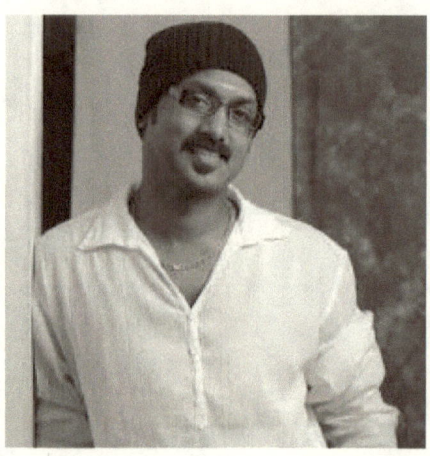

It was a sudden decision from the family that they came forward to donate his organs. One of the kidneys was allotted to us. We called a few patients on the transplant wait list as we do for all cadaver transplant calls. We have to do multitasking in arranging these transplants and every step needs to be accurate.

We always discuss with end-stage kidney disease patients regarding cadaver transplantation who don't have a suitable living donor.

A young patient who was on dialysis for more than two years and was on the wait list got the kidney. A successfully functioning kidney after the cadaver transplant was rejoicing for the patient, family and Nephrologist alike.

What is brain death? How does it happen?

Any disease, injury or trauma involving the brain if severe may cause the brain to lose all its functions. The blood flow will be normal, but the neurons are dead. As the blood flow is intact and the heart is pumping well, all other organs including the kidneys, liver, lungs and heart will be functioning appropriately. Few tests can identify the brain dead victims.

What causes brain death?

- Trauma causing brain injury
- Blockage or rupture of blood vessels of the brain (stroke)
- Oxygen deprivation to the brain

Are coma and brain death different?

In coma, certain parts of the brain are functioning. But brain death is a state of inactivity of the entire brain. A coma rarely has a chance of reversibility. But brain death is an irreversible state.

Which organs are donated?

Two kidneys can be donated to two end-stage kidney disease patients. The liver, heart, lungs, cornea and skin can also be used for the needy.

How to get kidney donations from brain dead?

Every country and state has laid down certain rules for organ donation after brain death. If a person has end-stage kidney disease and is initiated on dialysis, the patient is eligible for registration in the renal transplant wait list.

One has to register in the authorised hospital. The donor will be matched according to the blood group. Once the brain dead donation is feasible the patients will be called according to the seniority in the wait list. Cross-matching tests will be carried out and transplantation will proceed.

What measures the patient should take after cadaver transplantation?

Usually, the same kind of drugs and precautions for living donor transplantation need to be done.

PART 3

What You Eat Matters!

The Story of Salt

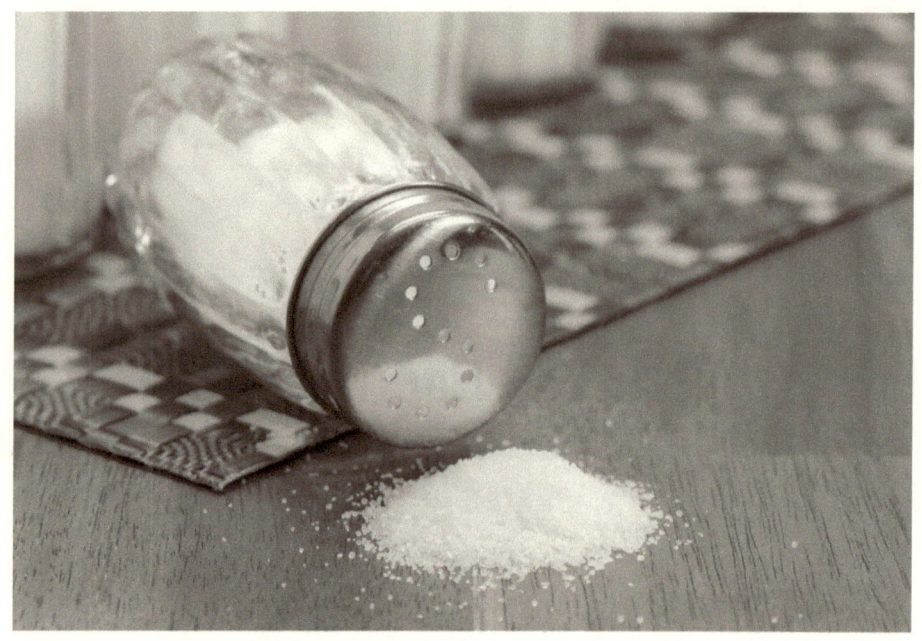

"Pepper and salt are indispensable in a delicious meal but if they dominate other ingredients, the meal is ruined."

– Vincent Nwachukwu (Weighty 'n' Worthy African Proverbs)

"Cheese and salt meat should be sparingly ate."

– Benjamin Franklin

Salt is Addictive

Salt is definitely addictive. It starts from early childhood. It may not cause any problem in childhood but the taste buds are adapted to it. When one is genetically or ethnically more prone to chronic diseases and if it is difficult to wean the taste buds, it becomes a problem.

Nevertheless salt is an essential nutrient and paramount for maintaining the mineral balance across the cells. It is present in every human cell, tissue, blood and fluids.

Humans are adapted to salt conservation and not salt excretion. As civilisations evolved, the kidneys learnt slowly to dispose of the excess salt but not to the extent of the quantity that the modern human being consumes.

The current salt intake is 10 to 20 times more than it was 5000 years ago. The blood pressure has to be raised to dispose of the excess salt via the kidneys.

The story and life of Yanamomi tribes will illustrate the importance of salt.

This Yanamomi tribe habitat the amazon region occupying Northern Brazil and Southern Venezuela, an area spanning a massive two hundred and sixty thousand square kilometres. The tribes form a total of around 35000 population. They lived a life akin to a palaeolithic era and their ancestors are traced back to more than 1500 years.

They were entirely dependent on meat, seafood and plants for survival and lived in a thatched house. Their average blood pressure was 90/60 mm Hg and their average salt intake was under 2 grams a day. Chronic diseases were virtually unknown in this group.

In late 1980, there were news that there are a lot of gold mines in that area and was intruded by outsiders. Outsiders socialised with the tribes. Their food habits changed, excess salt came into their diets and their lifestyle too changed. They are now burdened with a host of diseases like hypertension, kidney disease and cardiac ailments.

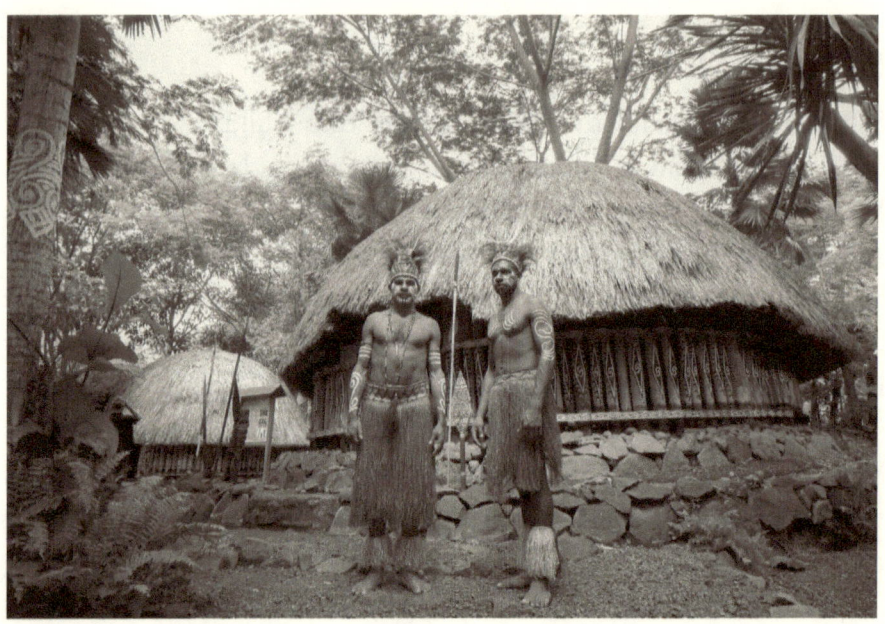

Rock Salt

All major rock salt deposits originated from the evaporation of seawater at some time during the geologic past. The Himalayan rock salt which we now use is mostly mined from Pakistan. There is no scientific proof that rock salt is healthier as some propagate. It contains few added minerals including potassium and trace elements but nevertheless are nutritionally relevant.

Recommendations are ignored

As per the World Health Organization, the recommended salt intake per day is less than 5 grams which amounts to two grams of sodium.

The average consumption of some countries

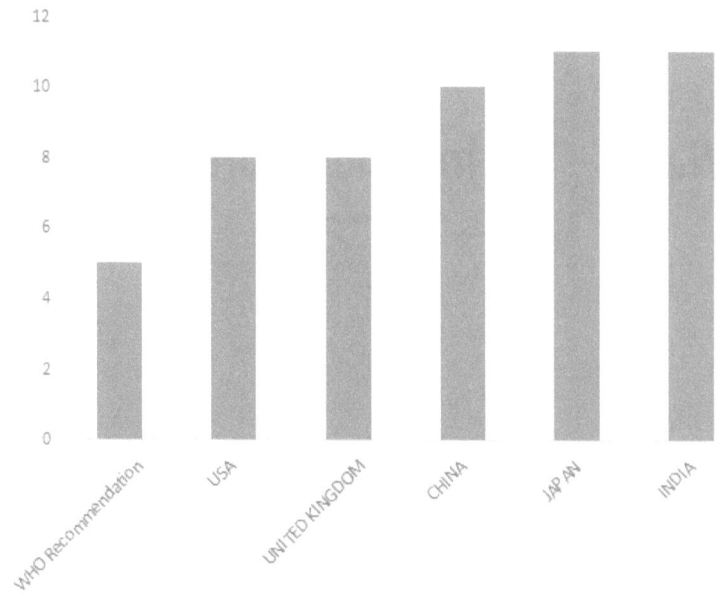

AVERAGE SALT CONSUMPTION PER DAY IN GRAMS ACROSS COUNTRIES

"A commodity of such importance should make us well and not ill. Use it sparingly and wisely. Wean your taste buds now."

Water – The Indispensable Medicine

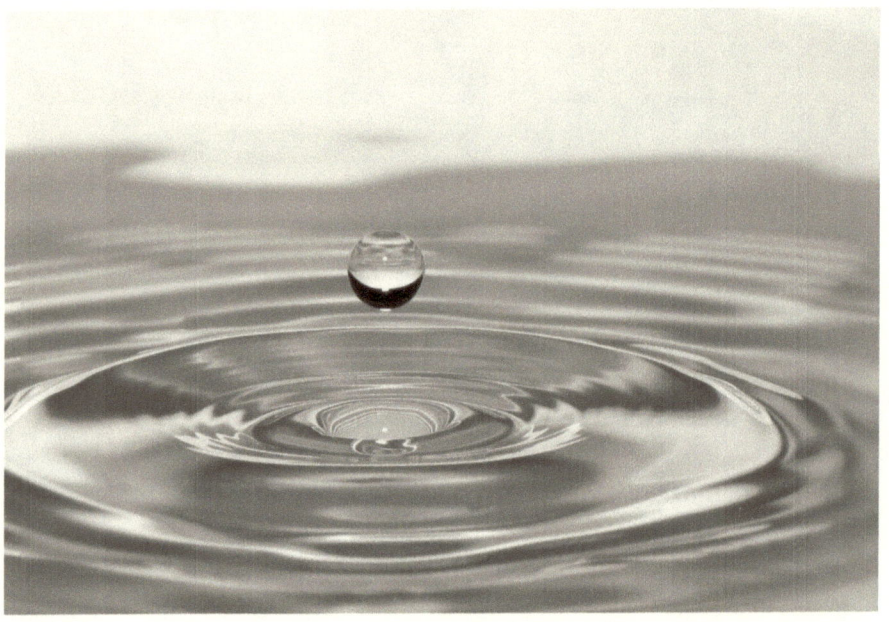

"The earth, the air, the land and the water are not an inheritance from our forefathers but on loan from our children. So, we have to handover to them at least as it was handed over to us."

– Mahatma Gandhi

Safe and Adequate Water is An Indispensable Medicine in the Modern Era

Our planet does contain over a billion trillion litres of water. But very little of that is safe to drink.

Nearly two million people die from a lack of safe drinking water every year.

In just 15 years, half the world's population would be living in areas of high water stress where there isn't enough groundwater.

Water and health

Water is indispensable for all body functions which itself is made of two-thirds water. Importance of water for kidney health is known but there is now overwhelming evidence that adequate water intake halts negative emotions like anger, hostility, confusion, depression, tension, fatigue and tiredness.

Unsafe water and kidney diseases

Twenty percent of the world population who are inaccessible to safe drinking water live in India and more so in developing countries. Drinking water is contaminated by heavy metals such as cadmium, chromium, arsenic, uranium and lead. They augment the already existing kidney damage and also have the propensity to cause new kidney ailment.

In certain parts of the world, there are epidemic proportions of kidney stone disease and kidney failure, the cause of which is the hardness of water and high level of metals in drinking water in those areas.

The Northern province of Sri Lanka is one such endemic zone where most of the people have no access to safe drinking water. The abundant use of pesticides contaminated the groundwater and the soil; most people had access to only contaminated drinking water. It is presumed that the environmental toxins led to an increase of chronic kidney failure in endemic proportions in that area. Most of those people with kidney ailments did not have conventional risk factors such as diabetes and hypertension.

After the introduction of purified drinking water in those areas, the disease tends to slow down a bit. This is the same case in many developing countries and this needs to be looked upon with greater resolve.

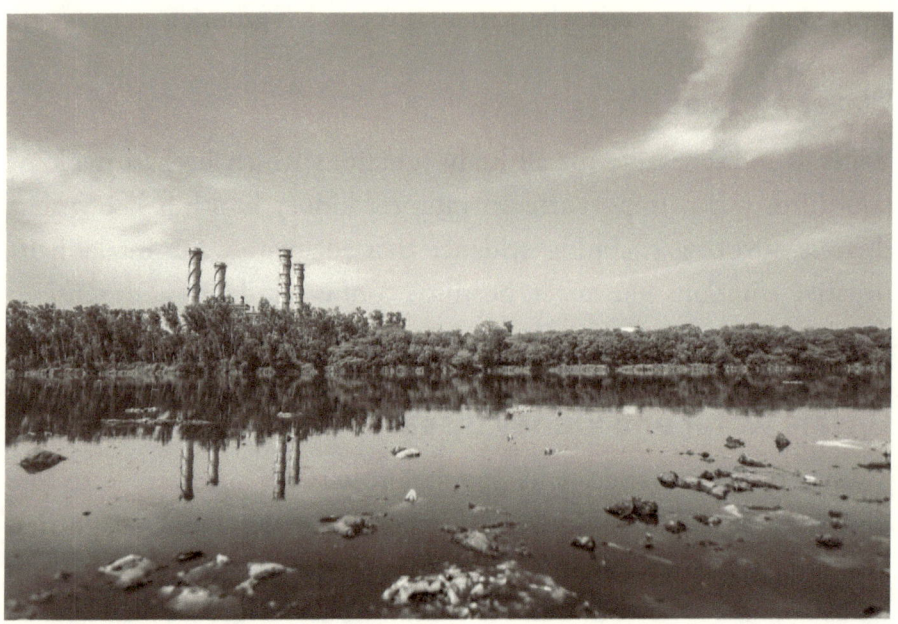

Drinking water and women

A unique problem in the underdeveloped world is that poor working women drink less water. Decreased access to closed space for urination makes them avoid drinking adequate water which in turn makes them more prone to kidney stones and urinary tract infection.

How much water to drink?

Water intake may have to be altered during fluctuation in ambient temperature and those involved in excessive physical activity.

Drinking a lot of water is beneficial to the kidneys, but if the same water is contaminated it would be disastrous.

Water in chronic disease

In chronic kidney disease and heart disease subtle alteration in hydration may alter the disease balance in a susceptible few. It is always better to have a check on the quantity in consultation with your doctor if you suffer from heart or kidney disease.

"Pure water is the world's first and foremost medicine."

– Slovakian Proverb

Diet You Need to Know

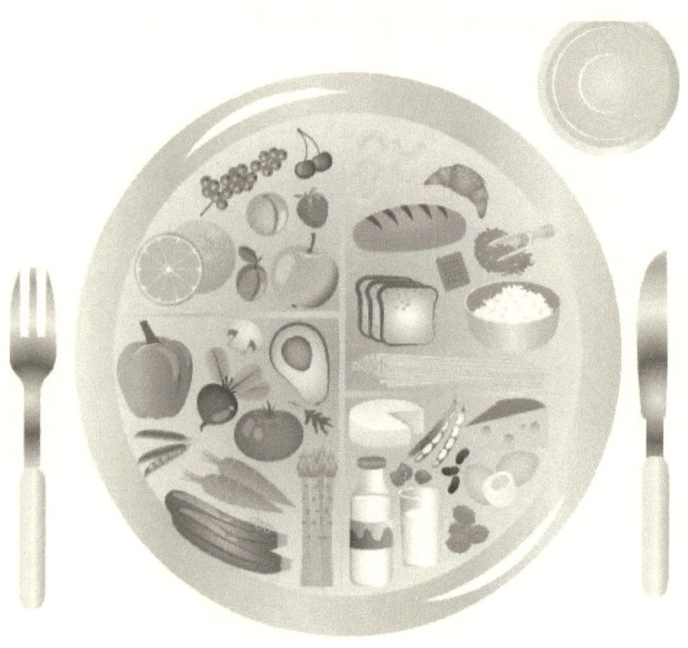

*"Let food be your medicine,
and medicine your food."*

– Hippocrates

> *"He that takes medicine and neglects to diet himself wastes the skill of the physician."*
>
> **– Chinese proverb**

The importance of foodstuff and its constituents, in general, will be discussed in this chapter.

Protein

The human body contains 75% protein. Protein is essential for the formation of muscle, skin, blood and bone. Proteins are also essential for immune response and fighting microbes. The proteins consumed are used up by the body and the waste products from the protein degradation are excreted by the kidneys.

Typical size

Amino acids make up the protein. When all the essential amino acids are present it is called the complete protein. The incomplete protein lacks all essential amino acids. The requirement of protein in the daily diet is about 50-60 grams (one gram protein per kilogram of body weight).

Complete protein:
Dairy, fish, eggs, steak, cheese, soy protein

Incomplete protein:
Pulses and legumes

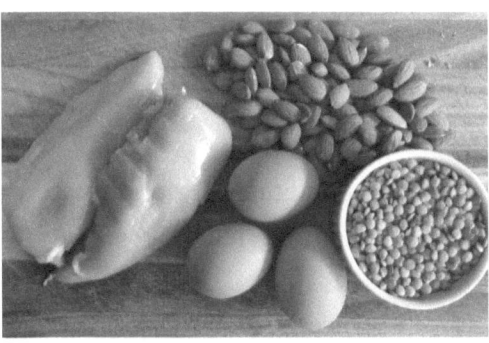

Fats

Like proteins, fats are also the building blocks of the body.

There are three types of fat.

Unsaturated fats are generally considered to be good for health.

Monounsaturated fats

They are found in high concentrations in

- Olive, peanut and canola oils
- Avocados
- Nuts such as almonds, hazelnuts and pecans
- Seeds such as pumpkin and sesame seeds

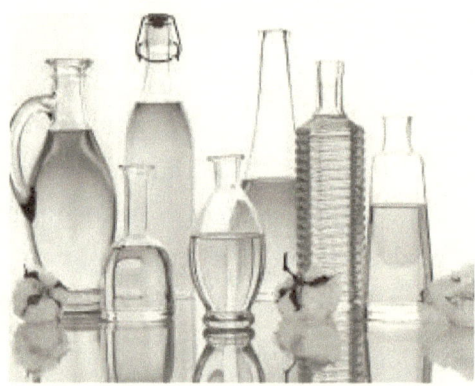

Polyunsaturated fats

They are found in high concentrations in

- Sunflower, corn, soya bean, groundnut and flaxseed oils
- Walnuts
- Flax seeds
- Fish
- Canola oil – though higher in monounsaturated fat, it's also a good source of polyunsaturated fat

Omega-3 fats

They are an important type of polyunsaturated fat. They have to be obtained from the daily diet as the body cannot make them on their own. Good sources are fish, flax seeds, walnuts and soybean oil. Higher blood omega-3 fats are associated with a lower risk of early death.

Saturated fats

Saturated fat is mainly found in animal foods, but a few plant foods are also high in saturated fats, such as coconut oil, palm oil and palm kernel oil.

All foods containing fat are a mixture of specific types of fat. They are not exclusive and hence saturated fats are not avoidable.

Trans fats

Trans fats should generally be avoided.

They are a form of unsaturated fat but are harmful to the body.

Trans fats are high in partially hydrogenated oils which are commercially used to increase the shelf life of the products. Hence it is found in *baked items, cakes, cookies, pizzas and biscuits*. Animal foods contain a negligible amount of trans fats.

How to avoid trans fats?

It is also formed when cooking oil is boiled above their smoke point eg deep frying.

It is best to choose a cooking oil with a smoke point above 400 degrees since most foods are fried at a temperature between 350 and 450 F. Extra-virgin olive oil (smoke point 410,) olive oil (436-468,) canola oil (400-475,) grape-seed oil (420,) peanut oil (440,) sunflower oil (440,) safflower oil (510,) and refined coconut oil (436-468) are ideal for use.

Sodium in food

Sodium chloride is otherwise called common salt. It is an indispensable content in most foods. High sodium foods are better avoided or taken in moderation.

World Health Organization (WHO) recommends 5 grams of salt (sodium chloride) per day which equals 2 grams of sodium.

Diets Rich in Sodium

Processed Food Categories
- Chips
- Pappad/pickle
- Cheese

Salt
- Baking Powder (Soda Salt)
- Ajino Mota
- Bakery Food Products
- Beverages
- Ice cream

Dry fruits
- Noodles
- Pasta
- Prawn/Crab
- Hot dogs
- Canned Soup

Foods with a Moderate Amount of Sodium

- Milk and yogurt
- Bengal gram
- Black gram
- Split gram
- Masoor dhal

Fruits
- Pineapple
- Mango
- Watermelon

Vegetables
- Beetroot
- Carrot
- Beans
- Cauliflower
- Radish
- Tomato
- Spinach
- Fenugreek
- Turnip
- Sprout Spinach
- Spices
- Coconut

Foods Low in Sodium
- All grains
- Red beans
- Horse gram

Fruits
- Gooseberry
- Papaya
- Orange
- Plums
- Pear
- Gauva
- Pomegranate
- Sapota

Vegetables
- Bitter guard
- Bottle guard
- Brinjal
- Cabbage
- Cucumber
- Onion
- Banana blossoms
- Potatoes
- Pumpkin
- Ridge guard
- Ladies finger
- Snake guard
- Sweet potato

Most of the vegetables have moderate or low sodium content.

Potassium

Potassium is another chemical in our body's cells and tissues. It is very essential for the functioning of the heart and muscle. Most food items contain potassium. When the kidneys are functioning well it can excrete a high dietary potassium load. Potassium levels may start to rise when the kidneys are not functioning optimally.

Consequences of increased potassium level in the blood.
3.5 – 5.0 – Safe
5.1 – 6.0 – Physician consultation is essential
> 6.0 – Dangerous level
Average potassium intake in the daily diet – 3 to 4 gms/day
Potassium restricted diet – Less than 2 gms/day
Your doctor will advise the amount of potassium to be taken.

High potassium foods

Fruits	Vegetables	Other dishes
Banana	Beetroot	Milk
Dates	Beans	Bread
Dried fruits	Black beans	Grams
Mango	Green carrots	
Orange	Greens	
Papaya	Pumpkin	
Pomegranate	Spinach	
Jack	Tomato	
Watermelon	Stem lettuce	
Cherry	Potatoes, Sweet potato, Tapioca	
Citrus fruits	Cape tuber, Millet tuber	

Low potassium foods

Fruits	Vegetables	Other dishes
Apple	Onions	Rice
Apricot	Radish	Coffee
Cherry	Broccoli	Tea
Pineapple	Corn	Pepper
Blueberry	Steamed carrots	
Cranberry	Green Beans	
Watermelon	Cluster beans	
Strawberry	Turnip	
Guava	Ladies finger	

Notes

Potassium is present in all foods, therefore, potassium intake cannot be totally avoided.

If the kidneys are functioning well, high potassium intake is recommended. This works well for blood pressure control.

Leaching decreases potassium content – How to cook?

- Vegetable skin should be removed first.
- Cut them into small pieces (1/8 inch.)
- Immerse in hot water and leave for four hours.
- Then rinse well with hot water.
- Cook with nearly four times water to the quantity of vegetables.

Some salt-losing form of kidney disease patients may not need to restrict sodium and potassium. Discuss with your doctor regarding your ideal amount of potassium intake.

Phosphorus

Phosphorus is found in large quantities in bones and smaller amounts in other tissues and is important for strong bones and teeth. Excess phosphorus damages blood vessels, heart and bones. Healthy kidneys eliminate excess phosphorus and it gets accumulated in the blood when kidneys start to fail.

The correct level of phosphorus in the blood:

2.5 – 4.5 mg/dl

Most protein foods contain phosphorus in variable quantities. The phosphorus content of meat is more absorbable than from plant proteins. The plants contain phytates that bind with phosphorus. Phosphorus in processed foods and beverages are also highly absorbed and are harmful.

Phosphorus is high in certain foods

- Dried beans
- Peas
- Rajma
- Chocolate
- Pork liver
- Chicken Liver
- Cheese
- Most processed foods

Reduce phosphorus intake in the early stage of kidney disease.

Fibre

Fibre is abundant in

- Whole-grain products
- Fruits
- Vegetables
- Beans, peas and other legumes
- Nuts and seeds

Benefits of dietary fibre.

- Dietary fibre increases the weight and size of the stool and softens it
- Helps to maintain bowel health
- Lowers cholesterol levels
- Helps control blood sugar levels
- Aids in achieving a healthy weight
- Helps to live longer

Non Vegetarian Diets
Pros & cons

The degradation of animal foods that are consumed causes high acid levels which are injurious to the kidneys. The better side of it is, it gives complete protein which is essential for the body.

Plant based diet

Are they useful in kidney disease?

It implies eating mostly whole grains, fruits, vegetables, legumes (beans, peas, lentils) unsalted nuts and healthy oils.

- Rich in magnesium and Vitamin K
- Avoids oxidative stress and inflammation

- Rich in fibre, vitamins and minerals
- Slows progression of kidney disease
- A good cooking technique helps to remove excess potassium

Presumed benefits

- Helps to maintain a normal weight
- Lowers blood pressure and bad cholesterol
- Reduces risk of heart disease
- Lowers risk for diabetes

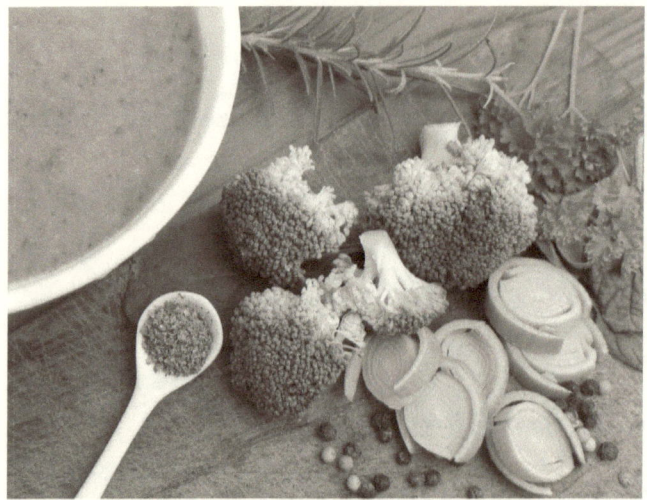

The Mediterranean diet and kidney disease

This is a typical diet of many Mediterranean countries such as Italy and Spain. It consists mainly of cereals, grains, vegetables, beans, fruits and nuts along with moderate amounts of fish, cheese, olive oil, yogurt and little red meat.

Of late there has been renewed interest in using the Mediterranean diet for kidney disease. It nourishes the blood vessel lining and hence is protective for most organs.

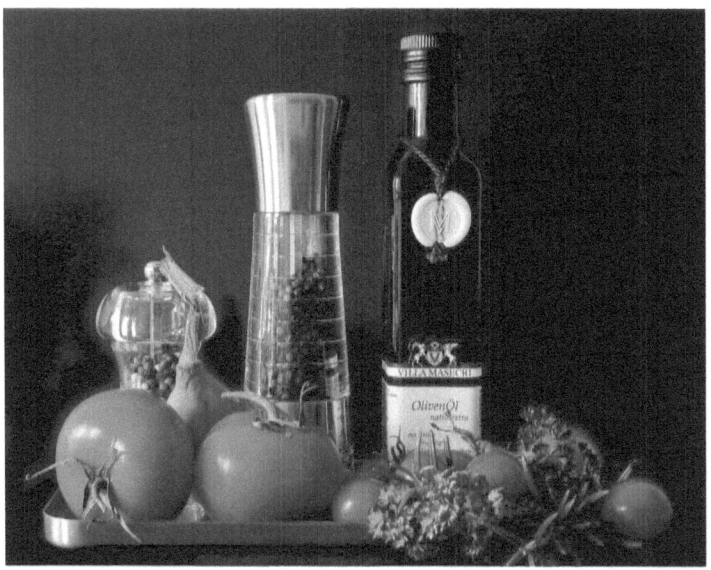

Are there enough calories in our diet?
We get most of our energy source from carbohydrates. They are called starch. They fuel the cells and are the source of immediate energy.

Simple starch

Simple sugars are broken down in the body easily. They are sugar-sweetened beverages and high-calorie desserts. If you take them, you're more likely to feel hungry soon.

Processed, refined or added sugars that do not contain any nutritional value include

- Candy
- Regular (non-diet) carbonated beverages such as soda
- Syrups
- Table sugar
- Added sugar

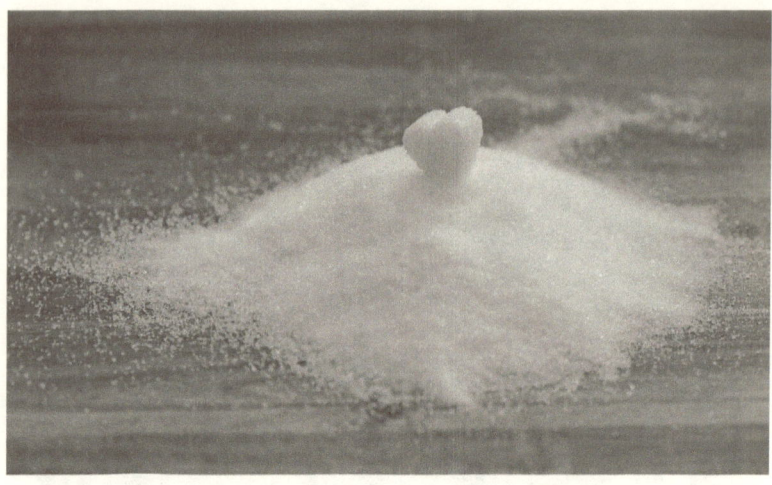

Complex starch

Complex starches are broken down more slowly, as with a whole-grain food. These types of complex carbohydrates give you energy over a longer period of time.

They include

- Legumes
- Starchy vegetables
- Whole-grain and fibre
- Fish – Salmon, Tuna, Herring

Glycemic index

Glycemic index denotes how fast the sugar increases in your blood after intake of a particular food. Intake of high glycemic index foods affects diabetes control and kidney health.

The laboratory evidence that carbohydrate-rich diets can cause the body to gain water and so raise blood pressure, just as salt consumption is supposed to do, dates back well over a century.

– Gary Taubes, Good Calories, Bad Calories

Regularly Used Foods	Possible Alternatives
Butter/Vanaspati	Cold-pressed oil
	Olive oil
Polished rice	Whole rice
	Whole wheat
Refined Sugar	Jaggery
Salt	Spices and Herbs

It may not be possible to follow all the dietary restrictions. As a patient, already burdened by number of pills and fluctuating appetite, one may have to try various food combinations before adapting to one. Identify what suits you the best. Individualise the diet for you and your family members. Adapt to the one that keeps your belly and mind relaxed.

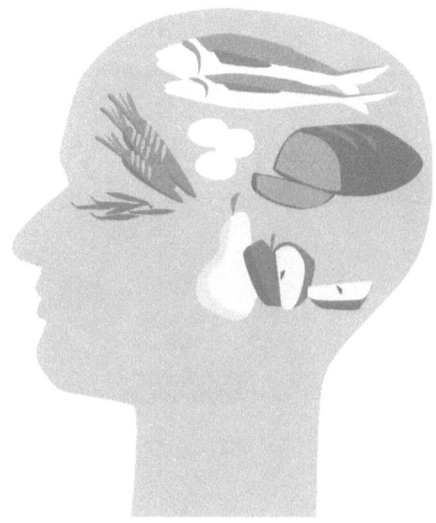

Diet in Diabetes and Hypertension Patients

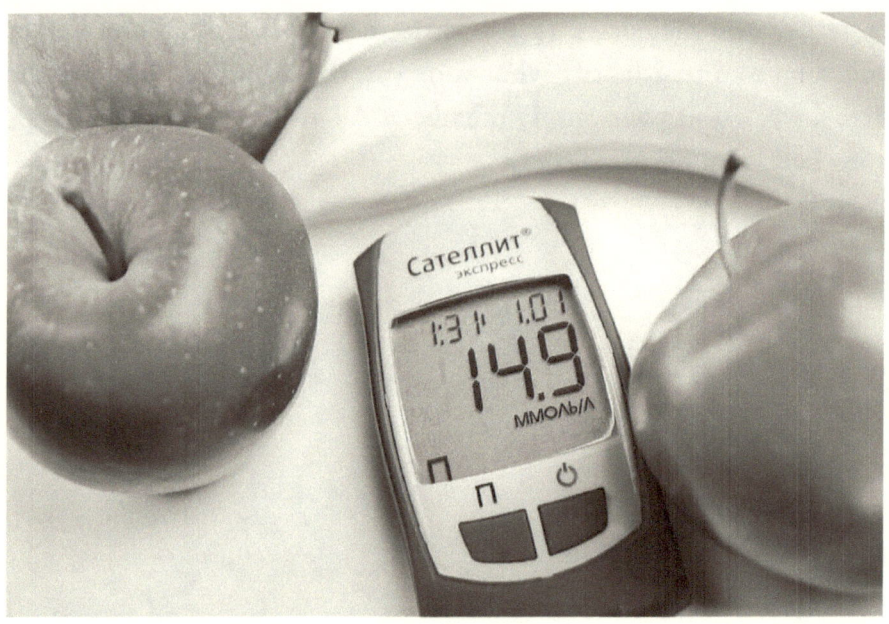

Diabetic Kidney Disease

Diabetic patients are usually loaded with dietary advice by their treating physicians. Few things are worthy of note in patients with diabetic kidney disease. This will help in a long way to prevent the progression of kidney disease.

Simple sugars

Avoid simple sugars and sweets such as regular pop (soda, soft drinks), sweet desserts, candies, jam and honey.

Beware of low blood sugar

With kidney disease, you are at increased risk of low blood sugar. Drug and dietary modifications when done should keep this fact in mind.

Phosphorus and potassium

Potassium intake may be tailored and adjusted according to your level of kidney dysfunction and consultation with your Nephrologist. If potassium is to be restricted citrus fruits, peaches, sapota, etc. are to be avoided along with vegetables like avocado, potatoes, tomatoes, pumpkin and spinach. Cabbage, carrots, celery and cucumber can be substituted. Limiting phosphorus and salt intake is a must from the early stage of diabetic kidney disease.

- Identify the foods which help you to maintain ideal weight which would help in multiple ways in managing diabetic kidney disease.
- Milk and non-fat dairy products should be restricted.
- The importance of a high fibre diet is well proven both in diabetes and kidney disease and is highly encouraged.
- Diet needs to be enriched with olive oil, fish oil and vegetarian sources of omega-3 fatty acids.
- Blood sugar control will help maintain fluid intake if you are on dialysis.

Hypertension – Tips for Good Blood Pressure Control
Weight Reduction & Maintenance

Try to change what you can do in the initial stage. Set a fixed target, start with 20 or 30 minutes walking and then slowly escalate.

Those who are obese can set a small weight target for each month. A small change in weight can have reaping benefits with regard to blood pressure control.

Persistent snoring in sleep hampers the control of blood pressure.

Fruits/Vegetables

Potassium intake should be minimized in many kidney diseases. They are particularly present in fruits and vegetables. But in patients with high blood pressure without kidney failure, potassium-rich fruits and vegetables are recommended. This can help lower blood pressure. In most leafy vegetables, potassium content is high and sodium content is low making them ideal for hypertensive patients.

Fibre

Studies have shown that high fibre intake lowers blood pressure. At least 30 gms of fibre should be taken in a day.

Best Food Categories for hypertensives
- Potato (High potassium and magnesium content)
- Beetroot juice
- Bananas (High potassium content)
- Flaxseed
- Skimmed milk
- Oats
- Honey

Foods to be avoided
- Sweets
- Sweetened soft drinks
- Foods high in sodium
- Red meat
- Fat – based food products

Diet in Dialysis Patients

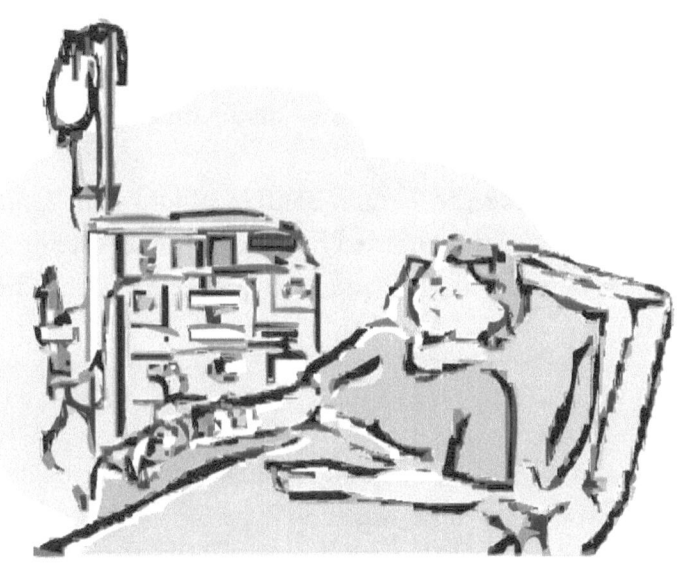

"What you eat in between dialysis sessions is more important than the dialysis therapy itself."

– Gloria Ann Jeff (Author and dialysis patient)

Proper diet forms the cornerstone to the well being of dialysis patients. It supplements dialysis therapy well. Remember that dialysis sessions will improve your appetite and you should be able to eat well.

Appetite

Decreased or loss of appetite is a major problem in patients on dialysis. Adequate dialysis will most often restore the appetite.

Protein

During dialysis, patients lose proteins. On hemodialysis they lose around 1-3 grams and during peritoneal dialysis they lose 5-15 grams per day. Added to this, inflammation causes more protein degradation.

For all these adjustments are to be made, intake should contain at least 1.2 g/kg/day of protein.

It is good to take the natural sources of proteins. Commercial protein supplements may be needed for a few patients who do not fulfil their dietary requirements. Soy products are high in branched-chain amino acids.

Fluid intake

The number of dialysis sessions and residual urine output determines the amount of your daily fluid intake.

By dialysis, the fluid balance will be normally restored.

Vitamins and minerals

Just like protein, patients lose vitamins and minerals during dialysis procedure and needs to be supplemented. The recommended intake is slightly more than the normal population.

Ideal weight

Your Nephrologist will determine the ideal weight. The amount of fluid accumulated beyond the ideal weight will have to be removed during the dialysis session. Ideally, fluid has to be restricted so that weight gain should not be more than 2 kilograms between dialysis sessions.

Tips to manage diet in dialysis

- Managing the diet well will have a positive influence on dialysis outcomes.
- A heavy meal just before dialysis initiation is not recommended.
- Nutritional supplements are best taken in between meals.
- Adequacy of nutrition will be reflected in the serum albumin value.
- Before going to bed, you need to ask yourself if you have given your body adequate nutrients for that day.

Example – renal patient diet plan (dialysis patients)

6 am:	Skimmed Milk – 150 ml (without sugar)
8 am:	Idly – 3/Dosa – 3/Idiappam – 3/Wheat Uppuma – ½ cup
	Sambar – 1 cup
10 am:	Vegetable Salad – 1 cup (Cucumber)
	Fruit – 100g (Apple/Guava/Papaya)
12.30 pm:	Rice – 1cup (Raw weight – 100g)/Chapatthi – 3
	Sambar – 1 cup/Dhal – ½ cup
	Egg White – 2 Nos or Boiled Fish – 2 small pieces
	Vegetable Porial – ½ cup, Curd – 1cup (50ml)
4 pm:	Skimmed Milk – 150 ml (without sugar)
	Whole Pulses – ½ cup
7.30 pm:	Idly – 3/Dosa – 2/Idiappam – 3/Wheat Uppuma – ½ cup
	Sambar – 1 cup/Dal – 1/2cup
10.30 pm:	Skimmed Milk – 150ml (without sugar)
	Total Calories: 1800kcal/day
	Total protein: 75gm/day

> *"Dialysis without proper diet is like fighting the enemy without armour."*

Diet in Kidney Stone Disease

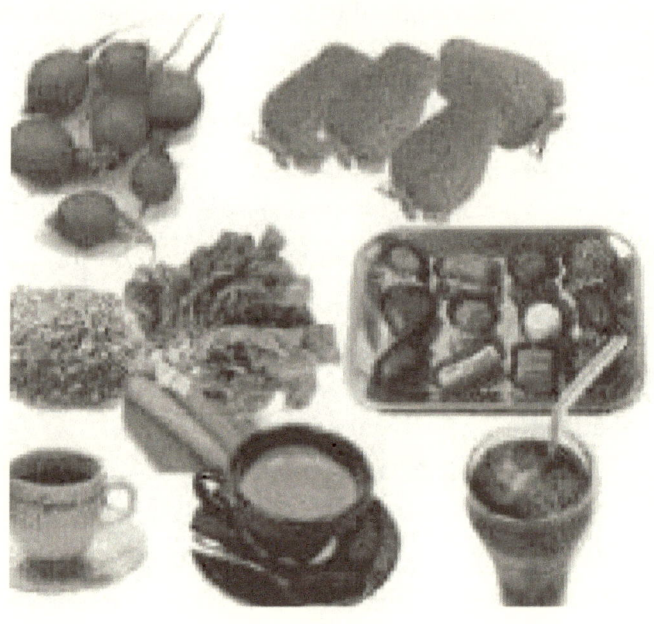

How to Prevent Kidney Stones

Drink at least three litres of water daily – Reduces stone formation by 90%.

Water and other fluids should be consumed in frequent intervals. Due to hormonal changes, during the night time, the concentration of urine increases and favours mineral deposition and subsequent stone formation in the kidney. So, it is imperative to drink a lot of water during bedtime.

Reduce Salt Intake

This prevents excessive calcium excretion as well as its deposition in the urinary tract. Salt restriction (less than 5 grams/day) is a must in stone formers.

Avoid Meat

High meat intake increases the formation of excess acid. This makes the urine acidic. This will increase the chance of developing stones.

Foods to Avoid in general in stone formers
- Refined sugars
- Dried fruits
- Grapes
- Peanuts
- Cashew nuts
- Chocolate
- Spinach
- Ladies finger
- Beetroot
- Sweet potato
- Frequent tea intake

What are the most common recommended foods for people with kidney stones?

These types of foods decrease mineral deposition in the kidneys. These can be taken in more than usual quantities.

- Banana Stem
- Ginger
- Gooseberry
- Ridge guard
- Cucumber
- Radish
- Consume foods high in fibre – 30 grams/day
- Calcium should be consumed in correct proportions
- Lemon juice – High in citric acid and prevents stone formation
- In general plenty of vegetables and fruits (at least 2 bowls) are recommended in stone formers

The exact diet also depends on the type of stone which is identified by stone or urine analysis.

Calcium Oxalate Stone

Calcium oxalate stone is the commonest type of stone. Those who have calcium oxalate stone should try to reduce the intake of the following foods.

- Almonds
- Peanuts
- Cashews
- Walnuts
- Chocolate
- Cocoa
- Beetroot
- Eggplant

- Tomato
- Orange and cranberry juice
- Soy products
- Rice and wheat bran
- Coffee, Tea
- Nuts
- Dark greens such as spinach

Uric acid Stone

Few persons have high uric acid in blood which is the causative factor for stone formation. They have to follow a specific diet plan as below.

Foods to be avoided

Seafood, duck, beef, pork, organ meats, mushroom, soya bean, liver, asparagus.

Foods that can be taken in moderate quantity

Meat and poultry
Breakfast cereals
Oats, Barley
Bread, cake, biscuits
Lentils
Spinach
Broccoli
Brinjal
Cauliflower
Green peas

Foods that can be taken in normal quantity

Egg white
All other fruits and vegetables
Cereals

Other general approaches for all types of stones
1. Lemon juice and lemonades are recommended
2. Avoid unnecessary calcium supplements
3. Take cereals and grains in the whole form
4. Potatoes if taken should be with the skin
5. Milk – less than 2 glasses per day
6. Weight reduction
7. Physical activity
8. Avoid hard water

"Discuss with your Nephrologist and nutritional therapist for the exact diet which would suit you to help prevent kidney stone."

Top 10 Super Foods

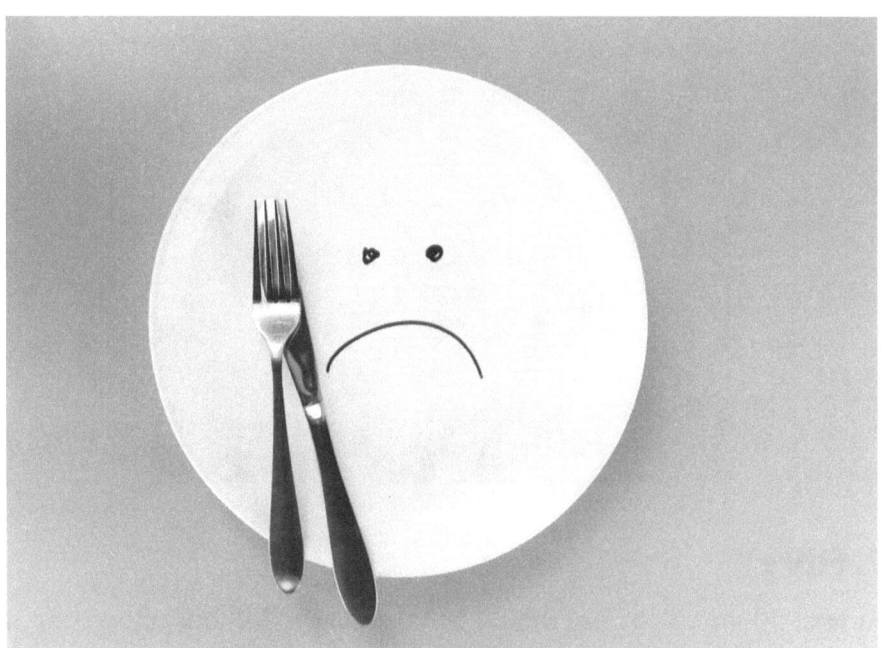

Few of the top foods suitable in kidney disease – Based on scientific studies

1. Green tea

Green tea is one of the healthiest beverages. Polyphenols are substances that are good for the detoxification of organs. Green tea polyphenol extracts contain a molecule called Epigallocatechin-3-gallate (EGCG) which is known to slow the progression of kidney disease. Though few suggest that it increases blood pressure, it should be taken in moderation.

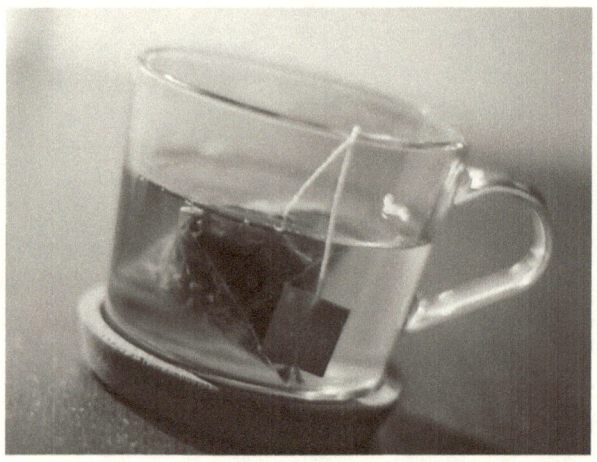

2. Fibre

At least 30 grams of fibre should be taken daily. Trillions of bacteria in the intestine produce toxins every minute that can be removed by the normal functioning kidneys but not completely by the failing kidneys. The fibre in the diet binds to the toxins in the intestine preventing them from going into the bloodstream and hence decreasing the toxic load on the kidneys.

The high fibre can prevent constipation which is otherwise common in kidney disease patients. They are also useful in the control of cholesterol and blood sugar.

The fibre content of common food stuffs.

Foods	Serving size	Fibre in grams
Split peas	100 gms	26 gms
Lentils-boiled	100 gms	8 gms
Oat bran	100 gms	15 gms
Pear	100 gms	4 gms
Whole wheat	100 gms	7 gms
Apple	100 gms	2.4 gms
Blue berry	100 gms	2.5 gms
Green peas	100 gms	6 gm
Most vegetables	100 gms	2-3 gms

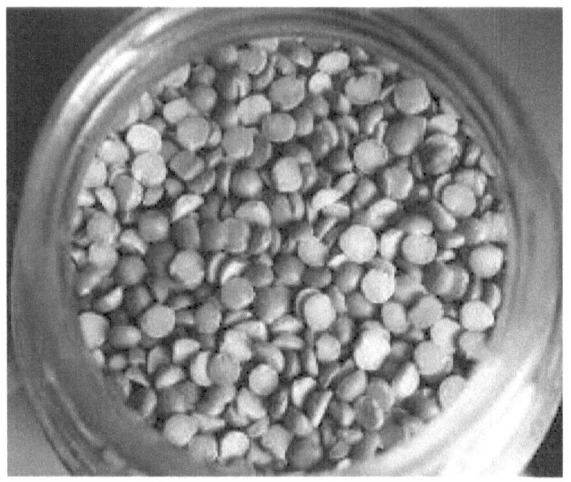

3. Garlic

They contain a chemical substance called allicin. The sulfur compounds in garlic is a good nutrient for the health of the blood vessels. It has antioxidant effects and is protective for the heart and kidneys.

The action of garlic on multiple body systems has been evident since antiquity and was widely used in ancient medicine. An ideal way to get all benefits is by eating a few raw and crushed garlic cloves daily.

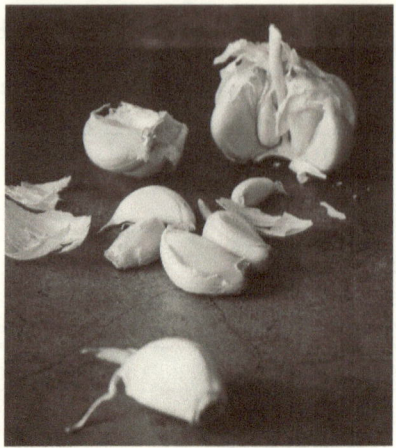

4. Berries

They contain phytonutrients, flavonoids and are loaded with a variety of antioxidants. They neutralise free radicals and prevent cell damage. Cranberries specifically prevent urinary tract infections. Potassium content varies with each of the berries.

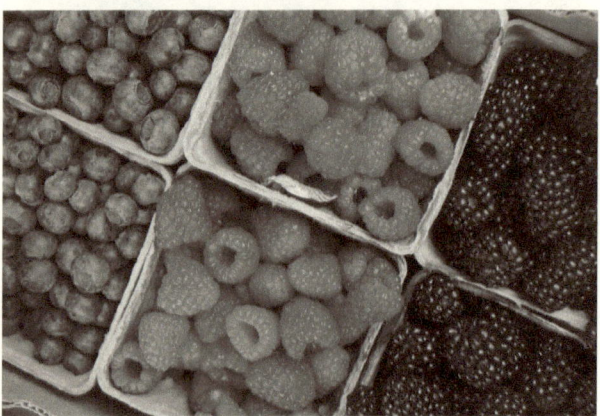

5. Egg white

They are an excellent source of complete protein, providing all the essential amino acids. Two egg whites contain 7 grams protein, 110 mg sodium, 108 mg potassium and 10 mg phosphorus. Phosphorus content is lower than the other sources of protein, ideal in kidney disease.

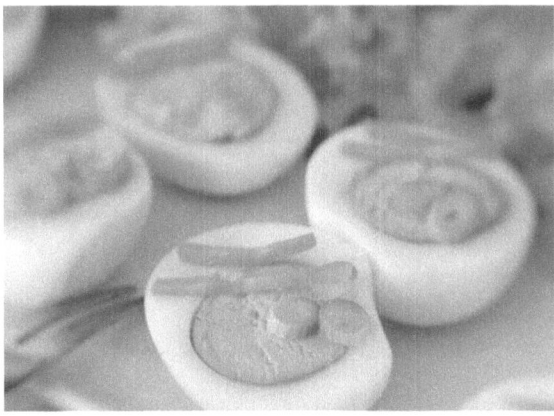

6. Fish – Salmon

Fish types containing high omega-3 fatty acids include albacore tuna, herring, mackerel, rainbow trout and salmon. Omega 3 fatty acid is an excellent anti-inflammatory molecule that is hard to find in other food stuffs. They have a high phosphorus content as like other animal proteins

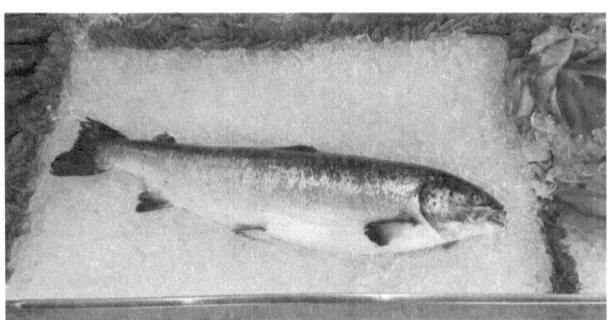

7. Onion

Good source of chromium, a mineral that greatly aids in the metabolism of nutrients generally considered best for diabetics. They are low in potassium and rich in flavonoids. They contain prebiotic fibres that help keep your digestive system healthy by feeding beneficial gut bacteria. It also contains quercetin, a heart-healthy molecule.

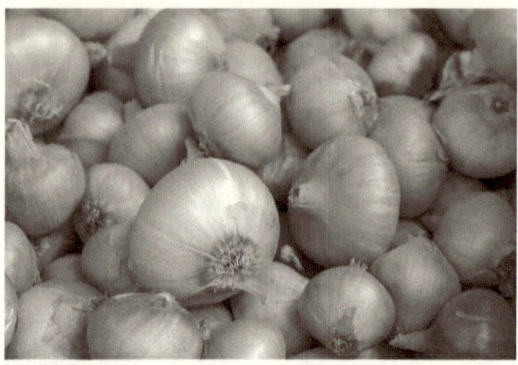

8. Cruciferrous vegetables

Cabbage, Kale, Broccoli, Cauliflower and Brussels sprouts are the cruciferrous vegetables. They make the diet less acidic, hence decreasing the load on the kidneys. They also contain calcium and are abundantly loaded with vitamins.

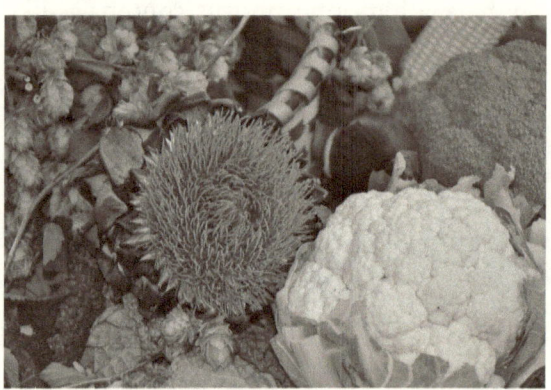

9. Few fruits to add and their contents
Red grapes

Half cup (75 grams) contains
sodium: 1.5 mg
potassium: 144 mg
phosphorus: 15 mg

Pineapple

One cup (165 grams) contains
sodium: 2 mg
potassium: 180 mg
phosphorus: 13 mg

Apple

Content per 100 gm
Sodium – 1 mg
Potassium – 107 mg

These fruits are alkaline which helps to counteract the increased acid load due to kidney dysfunction.

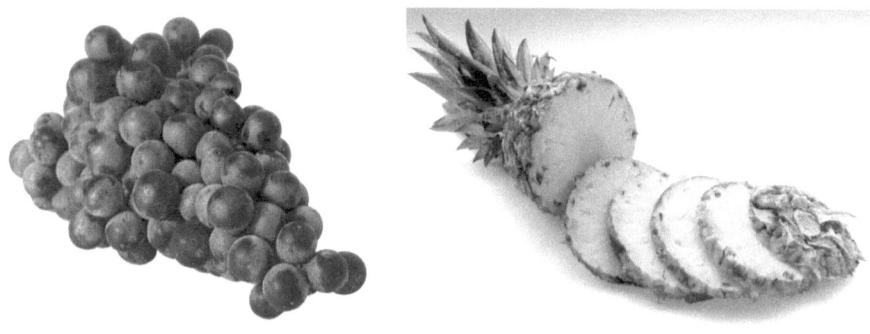

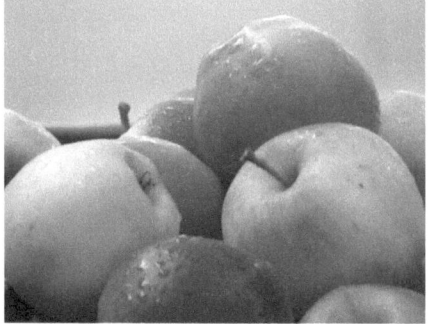

10. Radish and Turnip

They are high in Vitamin C, antioxidants and fibre with acceptable amounts of sodium and phosphorus.

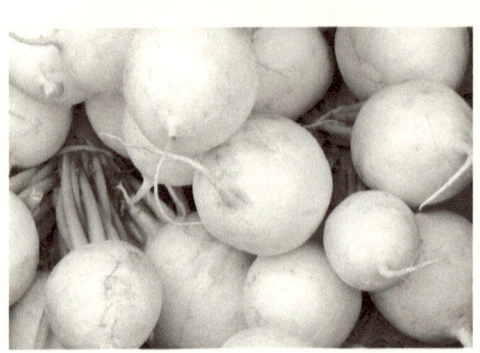 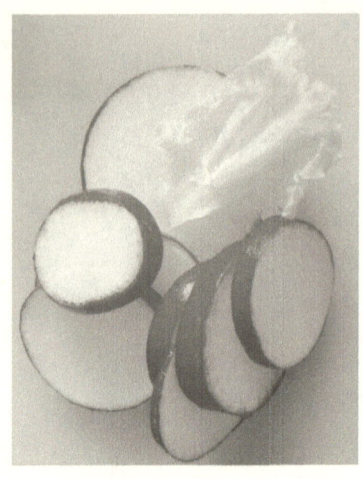

"One cannot think well, love well, sleep well if one has not dined well."

— Virginia Woolf, A Room of One's Own

PART 4

Kidney Disease Prevention

Exercise as Therapy

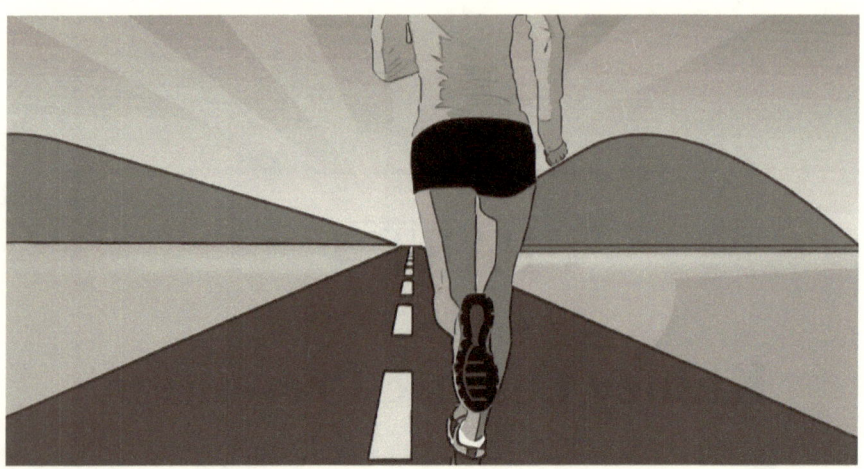

"It is exercise alone that supports the spirits and keeps the mind in vigor."

– Marcus Tullius Cicero
(Roman Statesman 106 BC)

"Exercising should be about rewarding the body with endorphins and strength. Not about punishing your body for what you've eaten."

– **Anonymous**

"The medical literature tells us that the most effective ways to reduce the risk of heart disease, cancer, stroke, diabetes, Alzheimer's and many more problems are through healthy diet and exercise. Our bodies have evolved to move, yet we now use the energy in oil instead of muscles to do our work."

– **David Suzuki (Canadian activist)**

One of my friends, a businessman living in my home town visited me one day. He asked, "All the doctors stress upon exercise and physical activity. Are they definitely useful? Do a fit person like me without any disease need regular exercise?"

I replied, "Yes, physical activity is good for everyone. This has been proven beyond doubt in various studies around the world. Even at a cellular level, it increases their activity. Exercise increases their activity multiple times through which every organ in the body enhances their power."

Some of the Common Benefits of Exercise

- Increases blood flow to all organs
- Blood pressure reduction
- Decreases mental stress
- Increases sleep quality
- Decreases cholesterol levels
- Increases bone strength
- Diminishes chance of dementia in elderly

How to do it?
It should be done along with daily activities. Try to be active throughout the day and avoid sitting for a long time.

Time: 30 minutes

At least five days a week

Initially start off with a slow pace and increase by five minutes gradually.

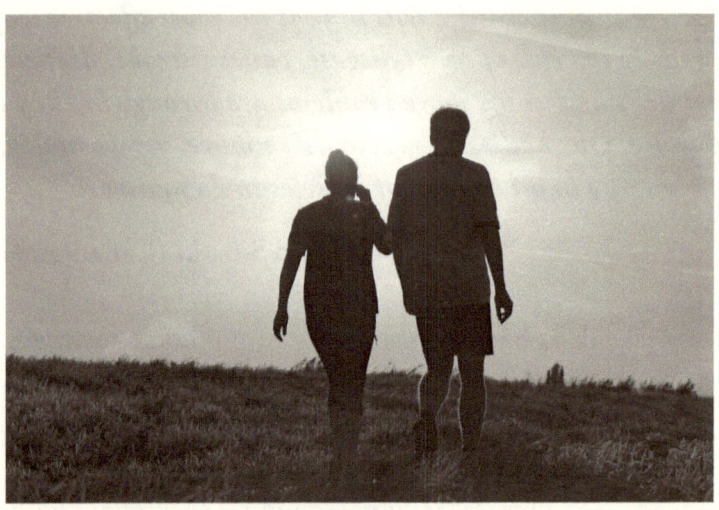

When should I stop exercising?
Stop exercising when you have

- Breathing difficulty
- Tiredness
- Chest Pain
- Palpitation
- Muscle cramps
- Dizziness

Benefits of walking

Easy to start and adhere to. Most muscles of the body are used during walking. You can walk indoors or outdoors. It is also very good for preventing heart disease, to which most kidney patients are prone. Some fluid may evaporate as sweat and fluid intake should be adjusted accordingly.

In many people with kidney failure, the muscles may be thinned. Exercise has the capacity for the regeneration of muscle fibres.

Worrying about weight loss?
Few patients worry that even with physical exercise they don't lose weight. Even without weight loss, exercise has reaping benefits. If one is obese, weight loss of about 10% of body weight has enormous benefits.

Exercise during dialysis treatment
Of late there have been interesting developments on the beneficial effects of exercise during dialysis.

Why reluctant to exercise?
A lot of people think exercise will make them tired. The fact is that even a little exercise will rejuvenate the mind and the body.
Ask your doctor which exercise will suit you. But start first.

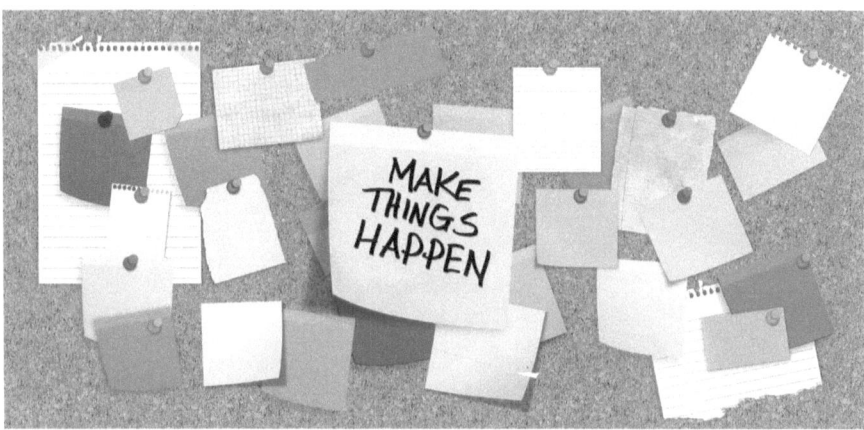

Yoga, Pranayama and Meditation

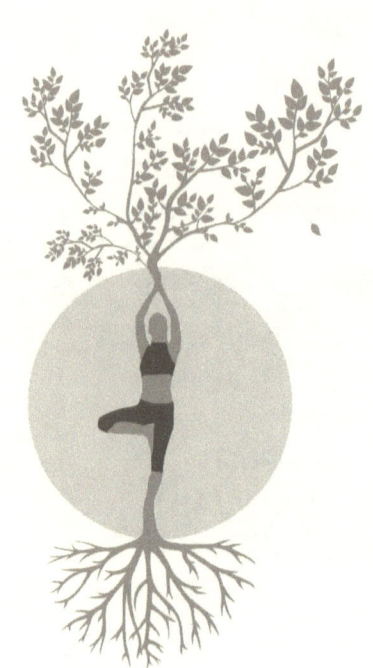

"During meditation, our breathing slows, our blood pressure and heart rate decrease, and stress hormone levels fall."

– Deepak Chopra
(Physician and Wellness Guru)

Yoga is being practised for over five thousand years. It is an Indian way of life.

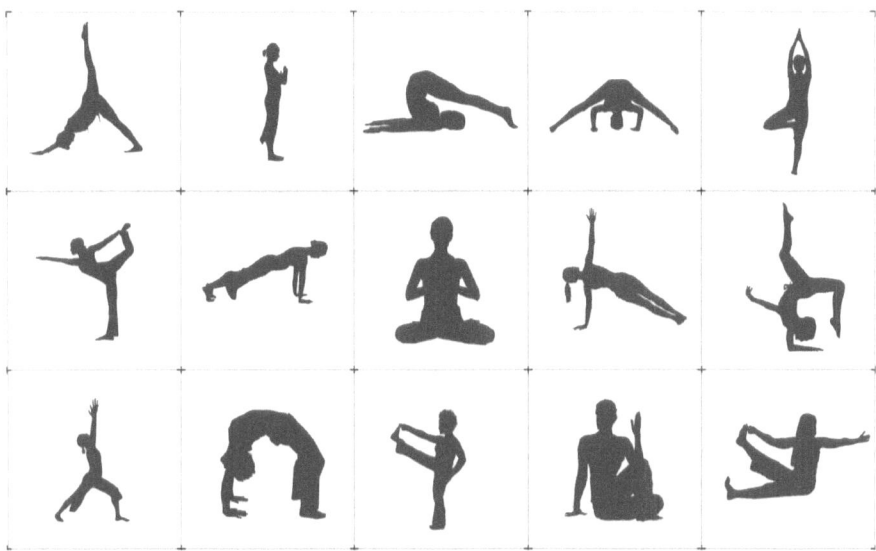

There is evidence that the sympathetic nervous system (part of the nervous system with excessive energy burst) is over-activated in kidney failure. This is a concern in uncontrolled blood pressure and progressive kidney damage. Yoga also indirectly helps to fine tune one's dietary practices.

It is beneficial for the disease in general and in particular to alleviate mental stress due to the disease.

It is good to seek the help of your doctor and Yoga teacher to practice it methodically.

Benefits of Yoga

- Peace of mind
- Regulates heart rate
- Decreases blood pressure
- Balances neurotransmitters
- Regulation of Brain Waves

- Giving a balanced lifestyle

Avoid asanas which increase heart rate and blood pressure.

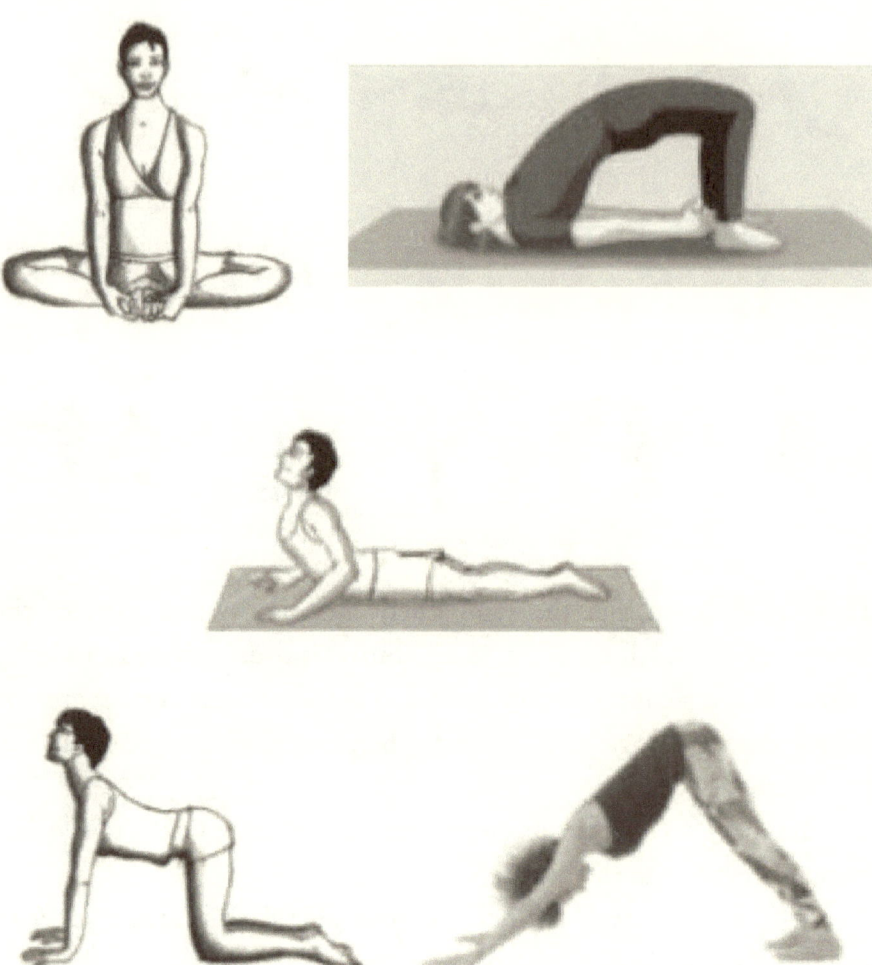

Pranayama and Meditation

These help to attain the highest level of consciousness. Pranayama helps to stretch the lung tissue and brings homeostasis to the body systems. Research has shown that they also help to reduce oxidative stress and a definite improvement in blood pressure control can be seen.

Heart and Kidneys

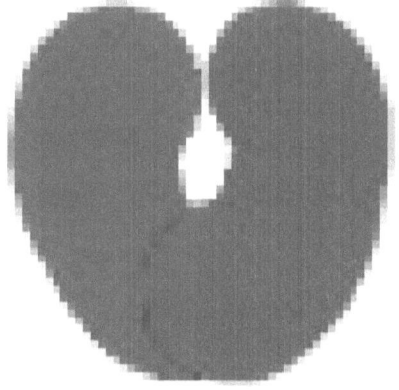

Kidney and heart health are intermingled. Both are vital organs in providing essential nourishment to every cell of the body.

Why do kidney patients need extra care for the heart?
There is a propensity for heart problems if there is kidney dysfunction. Diabetes and hypertension, both can affect the heart as well as the kidneys.

Salt
High salt intake may cause kidney damage directly. On the other hand, excessive salt increases thirst and increases the load on the heart. Fluctuations in other ions such as potassium and magnesium can also cause strain to the heart.

In end-stage kidney disease patients
End-stage kidney disease hardens the blood vessels.

In end-stage kidney disease, the cause of further worsening is heart attack and heart failure. In dialysis patients, the high fluid volume can put a strain on the heart.

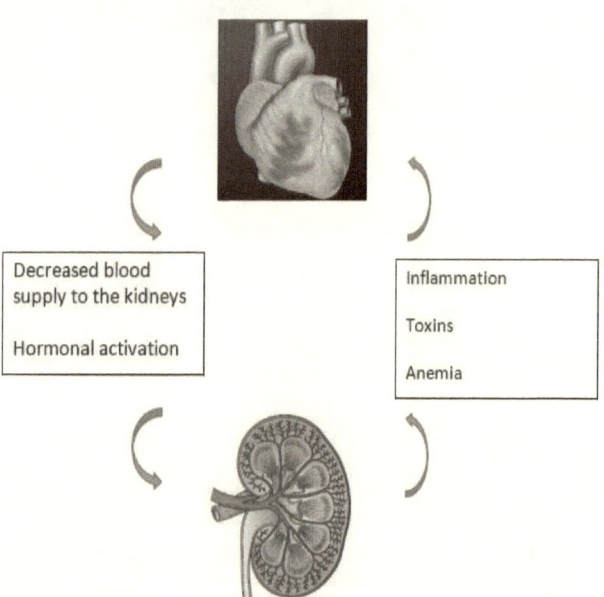

A cardiac patient needs periodic evaluation of the kidneys.

Prevention is Better than Cure

"No terrifying calamity will happen to the wise, who foresee and guard against coming evils."

– Thirukkural 429

"The doctor of the future will give no medicine, but will interest his patient in the care of the human frame, in diet and in the cause and prevention of disease."

— **Thomas Edison (1903)**

Remember

- Ninety percent of kidney function can be lost without any symptoms in a subset of patients with kidney disease.
- Complete master health check-ups should be performed.
- Urine examination, urea and creatinine are indicative of functions of the kidney.
- Examination of kidney size and its changes can be identified in an ultrasound scan.
- Calculation of Glomerular Filtration Rate (GFR) based on creatinine values will give an assessment of kidney function.

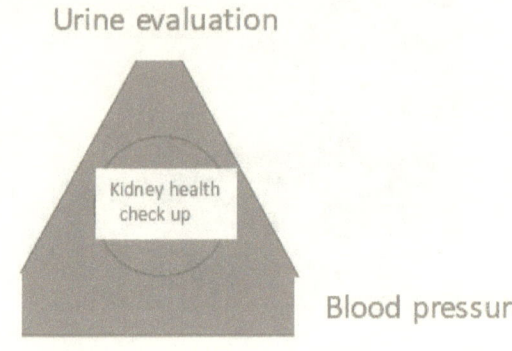

Early identification

Other Tests

Cholesterol

Just as cholesterol can harm the heart, it can affect the blood vessels of the kidneys.

Microalbuminuria

Testing for early detection of kidney damage.

HBA₁C:

Indicates our blood sugar control over the past 3 months.

Health insurance

Lifestyle diseases have increased due to a multitude of factors. Planning for emergency medical admissions and expenditure is a must if one wants to overcome sky rocketing medical expenses. Health insurance is a must for all. Discuss with your insurance company regarding the best policy that suits you. Almost all policies take care of dialysis and kidney transplantation.

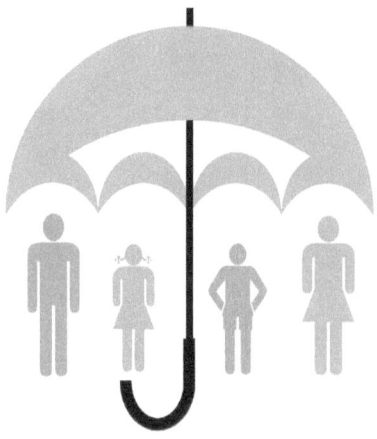

"I'm a prime example of the way kidney disease strikes silently. In my experience, you can identify and prevent kidney disease by simple urinary examination."

– Sean Elliott
**The legendary basketball player
Kidney transplant recipient**

Protect Your Kidney from Environmental Hazards

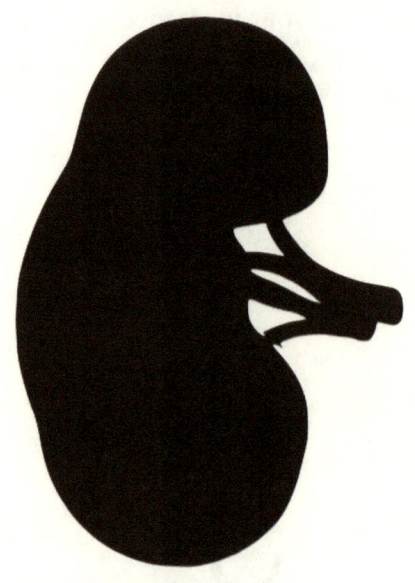

"We won't have a society if we destroy the environment."

– Margaret Mead

The environment is getting contaminated and the air is getting polluted all over the world. Industrialisation around the world has increased the disease pattern alarmingly. In kidney failure, new patterns are emerging. Though genetic factors are not modifiable, other simple measures will help in a long way to halt kidney disease.

Do Diabetes and high blood pressure can alone be blamed?

Diabetes and high blood pressure are common risk factors for kidney failure. Control of other lesser known factors will enormously prevent the occurrence of end-stage kidney disease even in patients with hypertension and diabetes.

The problem starts with the foetus

The vulnerability to kidney disease even starts in the mother's womb. Diet, nutrition, nutritional deficiencies and drugs taken by the mother have an impact on the baby's birth weight and subsequent kidney function. Good pregnancy care including good nutrition and foetal scan is of paramount importance in preventing some kidney ailments that may present years after birth.

Air pollution

In the United States of America and China, research has shown that the kidney function of people in cities with high air pollution is lower than in other cities. Pure oxygen parlours for the prevention of kidney disease are going to sprout soon. In India, the air quality index is three times higher than the upper limit.

Water pollution

We have seen how contaminated drinking water accelerates kidney disease.

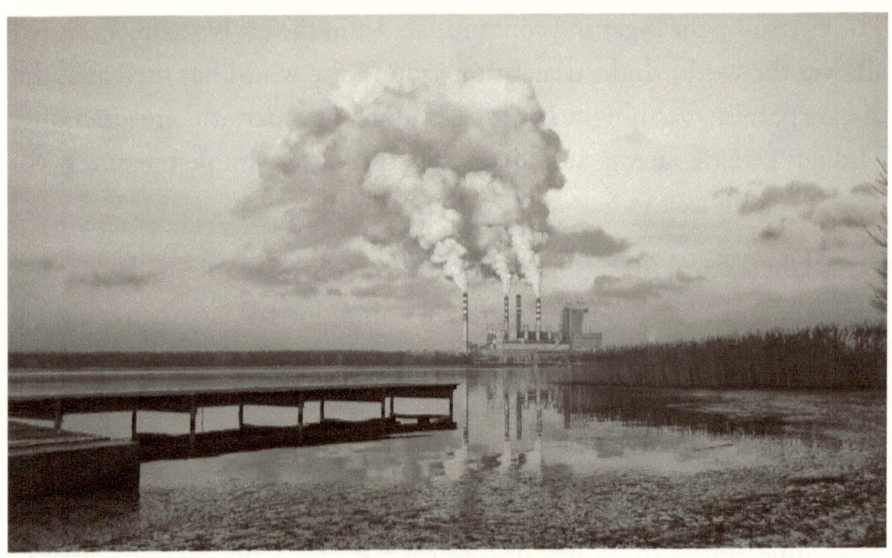

Kidney failure without a known cause

Diabetes and hypertension have been known in the past to be the leading causes of kidney failure. One of the most worrisome concerns is the fact that the incidence of kidney failure without a known cause (CKD – unknown cause) has increased over the past decade.

Recent studies confirm that approximately more than 20% of total kidney failure patients don't fit into a known cause. It is being a widely discussed topic among kidney disease specialists. Pollution due to the industrial explosion, excessive fertilizer, contamination in agricultural products and climate changes are the proposed hypothesis for this.

Comprehensive approach

Genetics also play a role in the onset of diabetes, hypertension and associated kidney diseases. But the above mentioned factors may exacerbate or induce damage in individuals who are already prone to kidney disease.

"The root cause of each problem should be sought and tackled."

Kidney Health in Your Hands

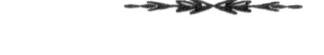

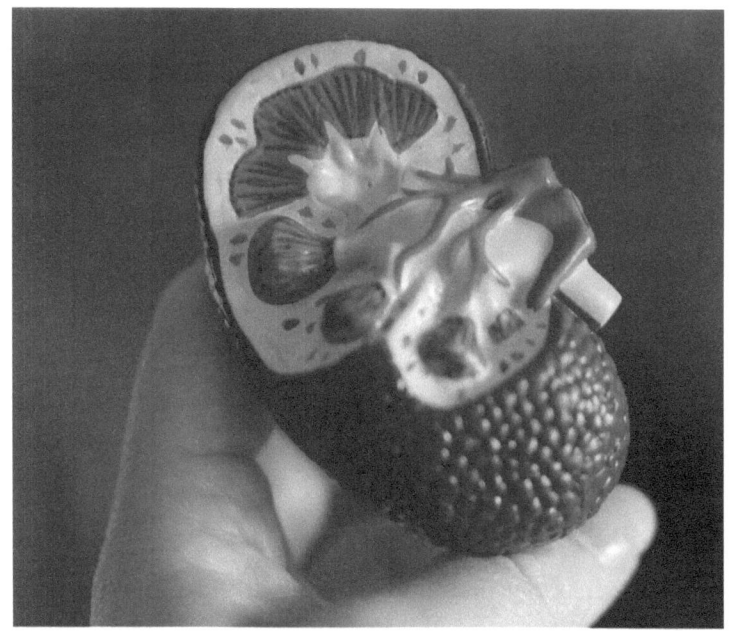

Simple Measures to Take Control of Your Kidney Health

Beware if you have risk factors

- Diabetes
- High blood pressure
- Kidney failure/Dialysis/Kidney Transplantation in family members
- Stroke/Heart attack/Heart failure
- Smoking
- Ethnic factors

Be watchful regarding the symptoms and signs

The previous chapters have dealt elaborately regarding the signs and symptoms which heralds the onset of kidney disease. The importance of a master health check-up in diagnosing kidney disease need not be overemphasised.

Take control of risk factors

Conventional risk factors like diabetes and hypertension should be under control all the time.

Don't smoke

Smoking slows the flow of blood to your kidneys making it difficult for them to function normally. Smoking also increases your risk of developing kidney cancer.

Diet

No diet is poisonous to completely avoid them. Moderation is best when absolutely healthy. Take the advice of a renal dietitian and Nephrologist right from the diagnosis of kidney disease.

Identify the real organic foods

It is proven that foods and drinking water contaminated with pesticides accelerate kidney disease. Take the effort to identify real organic pulses, cereals and vegetables and use them in your diet especially if you have certain risk factors. 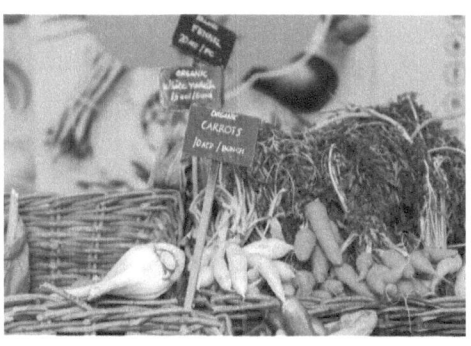 Many advocate a plant based diet for the same.

When do I see a Nephrologist?
If you have any one of the following

- Congenital kidney ailment
- Reduced GFR (Glomerular Filtration Rate)
- Proteinuria
- Kidney stones
- Acute and chronic kidney failure
- As advised by your family physician

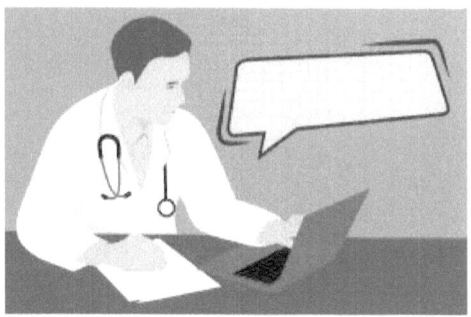

When you go for a Nephrology Consult

- Write down the important questions you wish to ask.
- Give details of your drug intake, duration and dosage.
- Go along with your previous laboratory reports.
- Get the records of home blood pressure and blood sugar values.
- Note your previous 24 hour urine output and inform the doctor.
- Remember to tell about the new onset of symptoms.
- Accept treatment with full confidence and clarity.
- Keep your health records up to date.

When treatment decision for kidney disease has to be made
Ask your Nephrologist
- What are the options available?
- Which treatment option will best suit me?
- How can I improve my health with the current treatment plan?

PART 5

Others

Kidney Warriors – 1

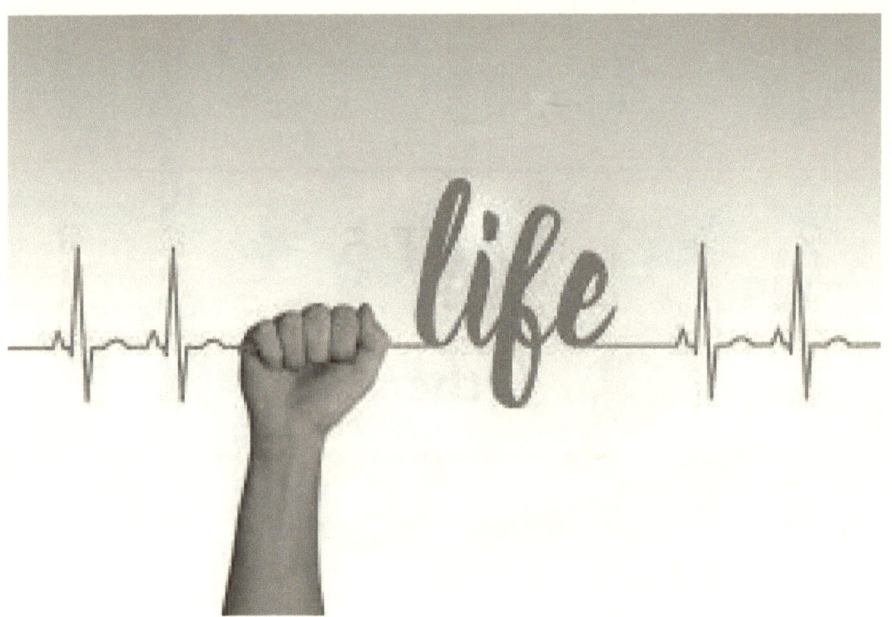

"Alonzo Mourning"

Many of you might not be aware of him. He was the prominent face of America's basketball team. He was crucial in the team's gold medal rush in the 2000 Sydney Olympics. He is also a seven-time winner of the NBA basketball tournament. He is Alonzo Mourning. All these happened after he overcame his end-stage kidney disease.

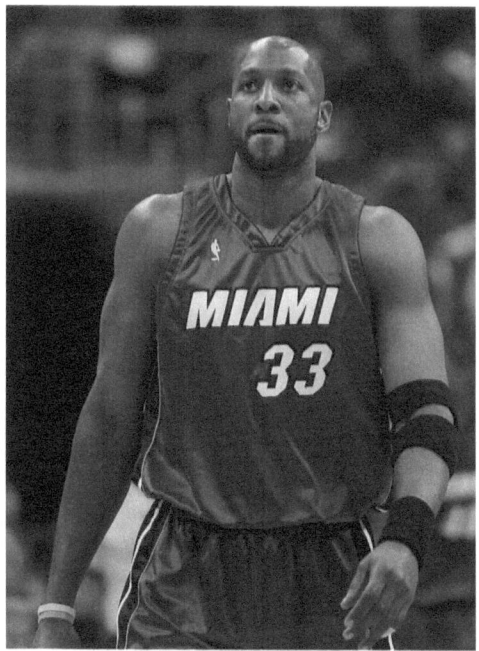

From an early age, basketball has been his life and blood. In his autobiography named ***"RESILIENCE,"*** he narrates how it was for him to understand kidney failure and how he overcame it.

"*Your life can change in a single instant, at the most unexpected time. One second you have a list of concerns, challenges and plans to deal with, in the next second that all seems trivial and God is laying down a challenge – a challenge you never saw coming.*"

He felt fatigued. His doctor ordered few tests which indicated severe kidney failure. He describes the moment he received the diagnosis.

"Many questions ran through my mind. It hit me hard. At the same time, everything was moving so fast and slow; my mind was racing and my stomach churning."

Breaking the news himself to his wife, he explains,

"So when Tracy saw me like that – silent, worried, head down, she knew there was a major problem. I told her what Dr. Richards had said. No cure. Dialysis. Transplant. Retirement. Understandably she started crying. She described her immediate reaction as being like a wounded animal."

Understandably a doom surrounded Alonso and his wife.

This was not before there was a *RESILIENCE* in him.

RESILIENCE to fight back the disease.

RESILIENCE to live a life of productivity and prosperity.

Alonso further describes his journey through the disease

"Together, we decided to face this tragedy. There is no other way to do this. You need to destroy something that attacks you. We must bring down the strength of the disease with the strength of our minds."

"You need to know as much as you can about this disease. Then we need to plan accordingly. And then we have to burst with positive thoughts. I have told others, Lord always has a plan. If this is his plan, then we must act accordingly. To overcome this obstacle, we have to put in the effort. It has always been my determination that I will win this. I talked to everyone about this disease as much as I could."

"Everyone thought my basketball career was over. But in the intellectual depth of my mind, I didn't feel that way. In those dark days, my self-confidence was tested in an unprecedented way. Even though I had a big physique, at times I felt like a small kid. But I was always determined to win over the disease. But for the kidney disease, I would not have had this amount of confidence."

"Confidence and faith gives us the ability to recover. But that alone does not make it easy. Continuous effort is required."

In 2003, he underwent kidney transplant successfully. His sibling donated a kidney.

Five years later, he played several matches and brought success for the team. In 2006, the NBA team he belonged won the championship.

"Diccon Driver"

Ironman Triathlon..

Hardest one-day endurance event on the planet.

The Ironman Triathlon is a dream for any athlete.

Consisting of a 2.4-mile swim, a 112-mile bicycle ride and a marathon 26.22-mile run raced in that order. It is a huge undertaking for anyone.

Body, Mind and Muscle must be toughest and fittest if at all you want to think of competing in this event.

An amateur triathlete refused to let kidney failure stop him from racing. With leg swelling, anemia and physical fatigue can one overcome these challenges in a single day!!

Diccon Driver did it with failing kidneys

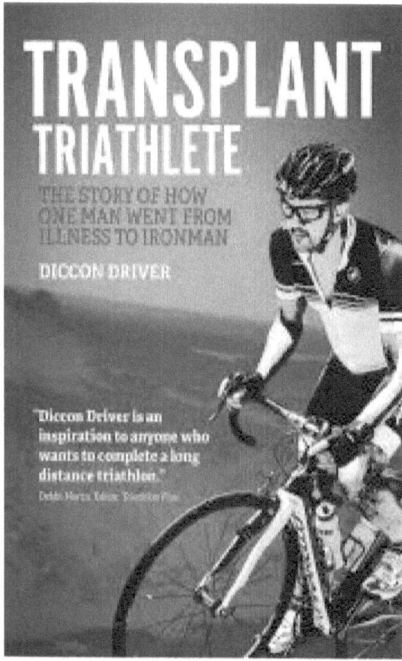

He describes his experience in his book TRANSPLANT TRIATHLETE.

He had been diagnosed with IgA nephropathy, a proteinuric kidney disease at 19 years of age in 1996. At the start of the national triathlon championship in 2012, the situation was not favourable for him. A few weeks before the competition, his kidneys were working at 25% of their capacity.

His legs were swollen and lodged with excess water. His blood cells were dwindling in number. But his mental stability was high at all times. His body went into shivers after the first phase of the triathlon. His thirst to finish the competition didn't subside. He successfully overcame the competition. Within a few days, his condition worsened and needed to be started on dialysis.

He was started on Automated Peritoneal Dialysis Therapy (APD.) Thereafter his younger brother donated a kidney. He underwent kidney transplant in 2013. This positive mindset of Diccon Driver is a lesson for every kidney patient.

Kidney Warriors – 2

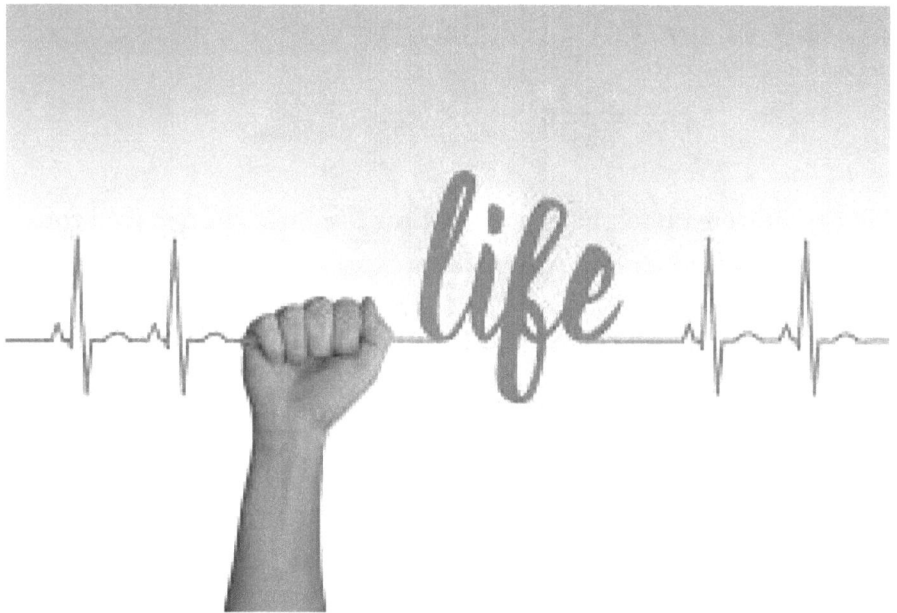

"Sahu"

I have a friend named Sahu who came back to fight his kidney disease after losing family members to kidney disease.

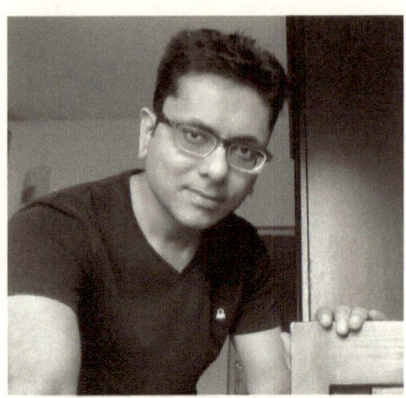

He has written a book named **"Fight for life"** which takes us through his journey with kidney disease. He starts as,

"It was during my pre-employment check-up at the age of 23 years my doctor revealed that the ultrasound scan was showing numerous small cysts in my kidney. He added that as I grow older these cysts would grow larger and may cause problems."

"He told me that my disease was genetic in nature and from what I told him it seemed to have come from my father's side since my mother was healthy."

"I told to myself, Let me not think too much about what the doctor said and let me lead life normally as before. I had put all negative thoughts in the background."

He then started taking medications for his blood pressure for a few years. During these times he took some high profile jobs in the IT industry. His kidneys grew to 5 kilograms weight as opposed to the normal of 300 mg combined weight. The disease progressed over several years and ended up requiring dialysis. He accepted and welcomed reality.

"No more running away from reality. Somehow I felt much lighter and better after this, as all these years I was scared of."

He says,

"I had ample time to plan and summon courage. I had a well stimulated mind to process such complicated information and derive a conclusion that would benefit me. I also never let the disease in my family or get me down and I stayed positive."

Planning the right mindset and courage can defy kidney disease altogether.

After successful transplantation, his creatinine levels trended down to normalcy and he finishes the book as,

"On the whole, my mental well being and satisfaction along with active life helped improve all my health parameters. I started spending time talking to patients referred by the doctor and from others who were aware of my experiences. Some of these patients came to my home to know how I had coped with my condition and understand what to expect from life next. It gave me a lot of satisfaction to hear that whatever I had to share could be helpful even a little in alleviating their sufferings."

"Kamal Shah"

For most patients, kidney disease and dialysis entail great trauma. Only a few see it as an opportunity to move further. God has separate plans for them.

One such person is Kamal Shah.

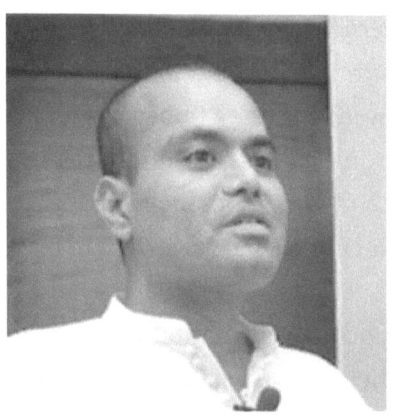

He is the founder of Nephro Plus, one of the largest dialysis providers in India.

He was diagnosed to have a very rare kidney disease Atypical HUS (blood abnormality causing end-stage kidney disease) which recurs in the transplanted kidney most often. The same fate beholds him.

There is no other option to be on lifelong dialysis at best. Nevertheless, new drugs are arriving by virtue of which successful transplantation is possible in this disease.

He encourages the belief that people living on dialysis can lead normal lives with quality treatment.

He has shared his experience through his blogs.

His illness started after he graduated in chemical engineering from Hyderabad in 1997 and was set to fly to the United States in pursuit of a future career. Just a month before travelling he began to feel symptomatic.

He recalls those moments,

"When nausea continued to persist for two-three days, I was a little worried about travelling. A family physician conducted blood tests and found out that my kidney function has declined significantly."

He then visited a Kidney specialist.

"A visit to the doctor and some tests revealed that I had Atypical Hemolytic Uremic Syndrome (AHUS) and would need a kidney transplant. I had to shelve my plan of going to the US and started dabbling in different kinds of treatment alternating with dialysis. I tried homeopathy, Ayurveda, acupressure, acupuncture over the next one year."

He then underwent a kidney transplant as a final resort.

Unfortunately, just 11 days after the surgery, things were not right. On the 20th day, doctors found that they had to begin dialysis once again because Kamal's AHUS had affected the transplanted kidney also.

He has to depend on hemodialysis and then switched to peritoneal dialysis when fate struck him again. While he was holidaying in Mahabalipuram during the 2004 tsunami he had a near death experience when the giant waves leaped into his room. Peritoneal dialysis got infected and he has to be put again on hemodialysis.

That was a blessing in disguise for him. He started writing blogs and he always felt that people on hemodialysis don't get the right quality of dialysis they deserve.

This made him start his own venture **"Nephro Plus" – A chain of dialysis centres** along with friends and well-wishers with a vision to enable people on dialysis across the world to lead long, happy and productive life.

Nephro Plus encourages the belief that those living on dialysis can lead normal lives. Patients here are called 'guests' and that's just the beginning of an endlessly comfortable atmosphere where they receive treatment through different modes of dialysis.

Now they have more than 150 centres across 22 states in India and also exploring overseas options.

His life only reminds us of the words of the famous German philosopher

Friedrich Nietzsche

"To live is to suffer, to survive is to find some meaning in the suffering. He who has a why to live can bear almost any how. When you stare into the abyss the abyss stares back at you."

"Vijay Shankar"

A journalist and creative writer living in New Delhi.

At the age of 65, he was diagnosed with kidney failure. He had to be initiated on hemodialysis. He summarised his experiences as a dialysis patient in his book «THERE IS LIFE AFTER DIALYSIS.»

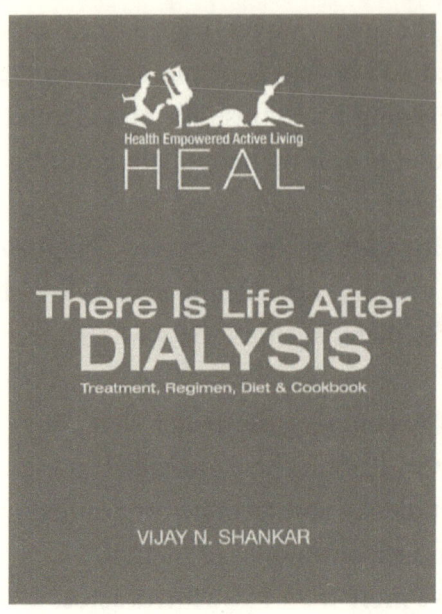

"I knew from the very beginning when kidney failure reaches its zenith, one can break down or can take a positive stride. The dialysis patient must create support teams around him/her. Luckily I got a good support team. You can avoid being a loner."

"People in good health usually face the first intimation of the disease in disbelief and denial."

He also resorted to many forms of natural and alternative therapies which didn't work for him. He expresses his displeasure.

"Many people in my position with the diagnosis of renal failure look around for alternative therapies. So much is at stake that you flap your hands and somebody drowning and try to get a foothold on hope. Also, there are numerous promise makers who offer guaranteed cures. Whether it is Ayurveda, Unani, Homeopathy, or a host of other natural/alternative medicines, the final truth is they just don't work as cures."

He was practising Yoga, Pranayama and Suryanamaskara for nearly five decades. Really these gave him energy and vigor to withstand dialysis. He didn't leave that habit even after the initiation of dialysis.

Every person with end-stage kidney disease should read this book.

Engaging Kidney Patients and Social Responsibilities

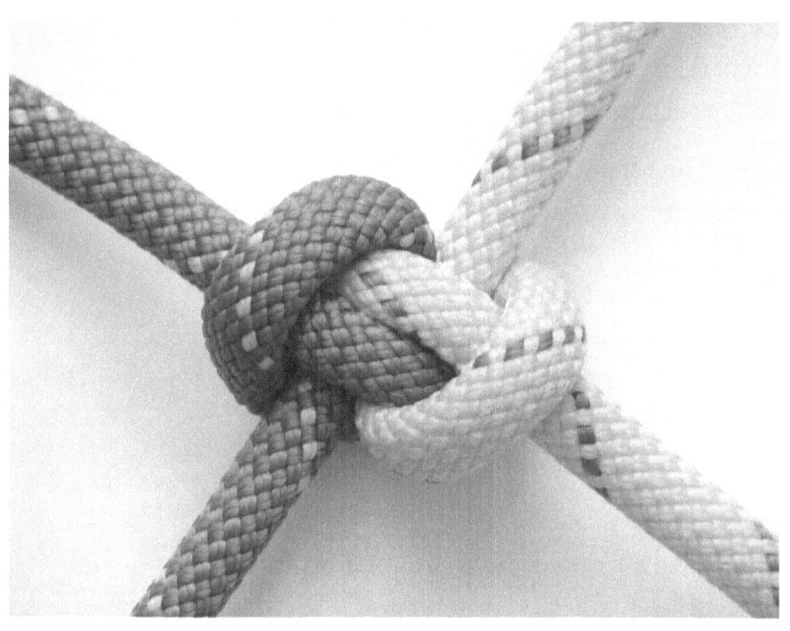

I am a kidney patient. Can I continue to work?
Even if your kidneys are not functioning optimally, you will have no problems going to a job if you are just on medications only.

If you are on dialysis treatment, you may need to spend four hours in the hospital twice or thrice a week. You can talk with your doctor and fix the treatment schedule according to your work pattern.

Even if you are a transplant recipient, you may need complete rest only for the first three to six months after the transplant.

How engaging in work helps?
- It will help your mind and body gain inner strength.
- Develops a positive attitude towards life.
- Increase your self-esteem among near ones and peers.
- It will help you feel productive.
- It is applicable to all, not just kidney patients.

If my near one has a kidney disease what should I do?
- If they are on dialysis, spend some time with them during the journey.
- Make them read books.
- Know about their complaints and specific symptoms.
- Note their diet and fluid intake.
- Take a walk with them often.
- Make time for yourself too.

Needs of kidney patients
- Social media channels to share their experience.
- Charitable organizations to provide a job for kidney disease and dialysis patients.
- Financial help as kidney disease incurs a huge financial burden.

Who all can contribute to the well-being of a kidney patient?
- The public
- Charitable organizations
- General and Family Physicians
- The government
- Nephrologist
- Family member

Frequently Asked Questions

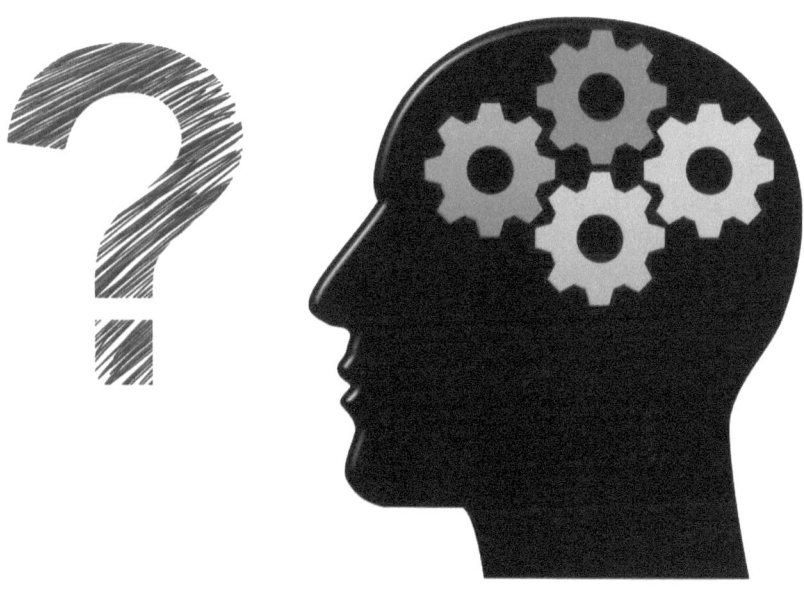

Does kidney function decrease with increasing age?
Yes, after forty years of age kidney function declines by about 1% each year. But naturally, our body adjusts to it and nothing untoward happens in normal circumstances. This is the reason why elderly people are more prone to kidney failure than younger ones during acute illness.

Is life possible with a single kidney?
Rarely one is born with a single kidney. The single kidney takes the function of removing harmful substances and body homeostasis is maintained. They need to have periodic monitoring and should avoid vigorous contact sports.

Even after kidney donation, single kidney takes over the complete function. They do not need any medications or any specific lifestyle changes after kidney donation. The risk of chronic diseases in them is almost akin to the general population. They need regular follow up with the physician.

Is kidney failure very rare?
No, a growing burden of diabetes and high blood pressure, changing lifestyle and food habits cause a high likelihood of kidney failure. Asian ethnics have a high chance of kidney failure. Overall about 10% of the world population is at risk of chronic kidney failure.

Does kidney disease always occur with symptoms?
It is an old thought. In most kidney diseases, there will be no symptoms in the initial period. The symptoms appear later and few are extremely asymptomatic until the final stage.

Does it cost a lot to know that you have kidney damage?
No, a simple urine test and one or two blood tests are sufficient.

Is it difficult to know about kidney diseases?
No, it is not difficult, and spending a few hours can help you achieve the desired knowledge and protect your kidneys. That is why this book is in your hands.

My e GFR is more than 60. Should I consult a Nephrologist?
If you have protein in urine, abnormalities in the kidney scan or abnormal urinary symptoms you have to consult a Nephrologist even if the kidney function is normal.

At any cost, if I am able to reduce the creatinine level in the blood, will the kidneys recover?
No, such efforts should not be made and sometimes they may be detrimental. Meet your doctor and take measures to stabilize your kidney function. Don't trace the creatinine level.

Is dialysis the only solution for kidney damage?
Dialysis is not the solution for every kidney patient. Discuss with your Nephrologist to know the correct treatment tailored to your stage of kidney disease.

My near one has end-stage kidney disease. Will he tolerate dialysis?
In end-stage kidney disease, there will be variable symptoms. If one postpones dialysis in those situations there is a chance of further worsening of symptoms. When required, dialysis and supportive medications alone will help regain health.

With very strict diet restrictions can I cure my kidney disease?
The disease can be prevented to some extent. After the disease onset, its progression can be delayed with lifestyle changes and medications.

Does sleep get affected by kidney diseases?
Sleep depends on both physical and mental well being which means you should have a hold on both of these to have a good sleep.

Once started, do we need to continue dialysis lifelong for end-stage kidney disease patients?
Generally, Yes. In end-stage kidney disease, very rarely around 2% of patients regain sufficient renal function to discontinue dialysis. Renal transplantation is the treatment of choice to replace the kidney function naturally.

Common Drugs in Kidney Diseases

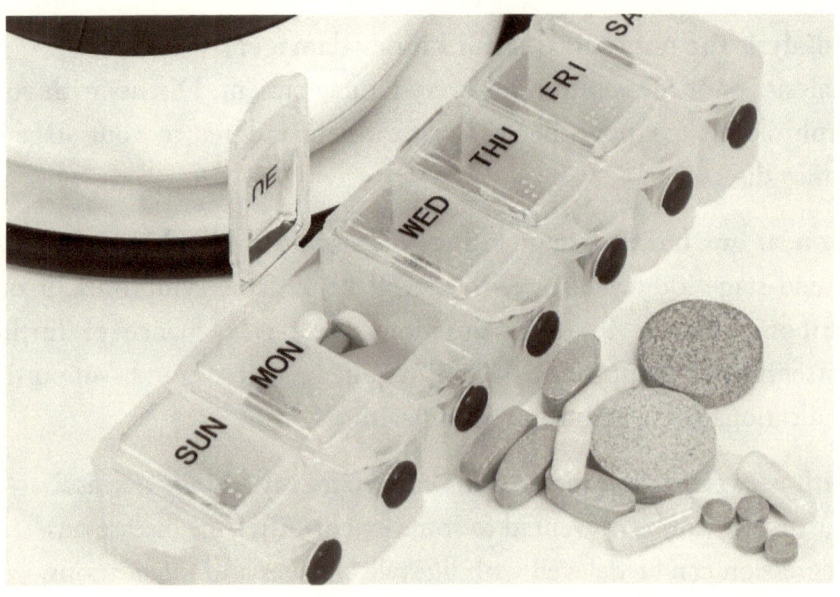

Diuretics

These are the drugs that push the excess fluid accumulated in the body and increase urine volume. They also marginally lower blood pressure. Ideally, body weight and levels of sodium and potassium need to be monitored at least for the initial few days after initiation of these drugs.

Blood pressure lowering medications

Most kidney patients have high blood pressure as kidneys play an important role in maintaining normal blood pressure. At times more than one drug may be needed. Some commonly used drugs are Amlodipine, Nifedipine, Telmisartan, Olmesartan, Losartan, Ramipril and Metoprolol. Few of these drugs also decrease the amount of protein loss in urine

Sodium Bicarbonate

This is used in all stages of chronic kidney disease in varying doses. It helps mitigate the acidic load on the kidneys.

Cholesterol lowering drugs

As kidney failure patients are more prone to adverse effects of cholesterol, they are more often prescribed cholesterol lowering drugs such as Statins.

Blood thinners

Antiplatelet medications like Aspirin or Clopidogrel may be prescribed if you are at risk of blood vessel occlusion (vascular disease.)

Iron and Vitamin supplements

Kidney failure patients most often suffer from nutrient deficiencies. These supplements are often prescribed to them.

Other drugs

Calcium supplements, drugs that bind phosphate and potassium in the intestine, Erythropoietin are the other commonly used drugs in kidney ailment.

Become an Organ Donor

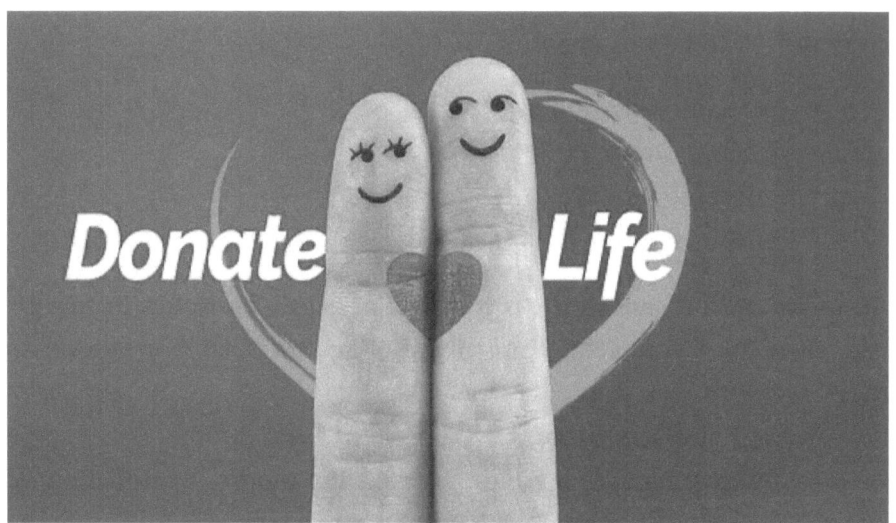

"You give but little when you give of your possessions. It is when you give of yourself that you truly give."

– Khalil Gibran

The global burden of end-stage kidney disease and organ failure is ever increasing. More than five lakh patients die of organ failure every year in India. There are more than one million kidney disease patients. One and a half million people have registered for kidneys and are waiting. But only about five thousand kidney transplants are done annually.

A brain dead person can give life to 9 people with various organ dysfunctions. Even if a person has registered for organ donation, it is the family who decides for and against organ donation after brain death.

It is thus necessary that everyone should be aware of organ donation.

Various charitable organizations are involved in organ donation awareness in India.

- mohanfoundation.org
- shataya.org.in
- giftyourorgan.org
- giftlife.org

An incident that caused the revolution of organ donation in India

The death of a young boy caused the organ transplant revolution in India.

It was a pleasant Saturday evening in the year 2008.

A young student, Hithendran asked his mother's permission to take the two-wheeler to spend some time with his friends outside.

His mother who refused initially then allowed him unwillingly.

When a speeding bus collided with his two-wheeler on the road, he fell down unconscious. His parents who both were doctors immediately arrived there. He was shifted to a hospital in Chennai.

Doctors told them that he was brain dead. Organs including kidney and liver were retrieved and transplanted to patients in Apollo Hospital. A nine-year-old girl with heart failure was given his heart.

The boy Hithendran's father Dr. Asokhan then said,

"My son has survived six.
He is not dead but is alive."

This incident brings back to my mind, the poem written by Robert Trust on organ donation.

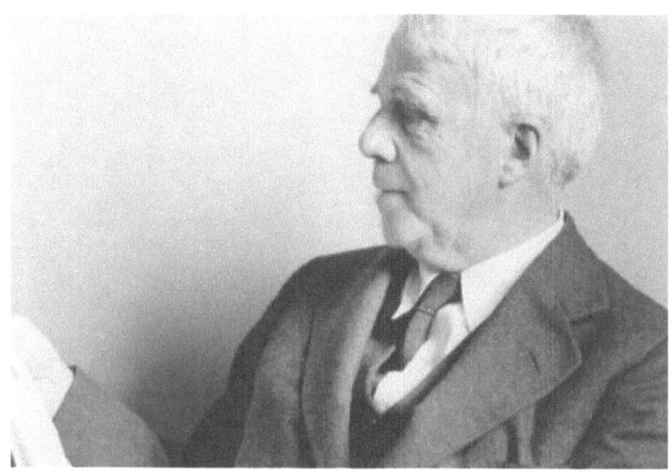

Give my sight to the man who has never seen a sunrise, a baby's face, or love in the eyes of a woman.

Give my heart to a person whose own heart has caused nothing but endless days of pain.

Give my blood to the teenager who was pulled from the wreckage of his car, so that he might live to see his grandchildren play.

Give my kidneys to one who depends on a machine to exist from week to week.

Take my bones, every muscle, every fibre and nerve in my body and d a way to make a crippled child walk.

If you must bury something, let it be my faults, my weaknesses and all prejudice against my fellow man.

Give my sins to the devil.

Give my soul to God.

If, by chance, you wish to remember me, do it with a kind deed or word to someone who needs you. If you do all I have asked, I will live forever.

www.ingramcontent.com/pod-product-compliance
Lightning Source LLC
Chambersburg PA
CBHW030930180526
45163CB00002B/518